Infant Feeding - Breast versus Formula

Edited by Isam Jaber Al-Zwaini, Zaid Rasheed Al-Ani and Walter Hurley

Published in London, United Kingdom

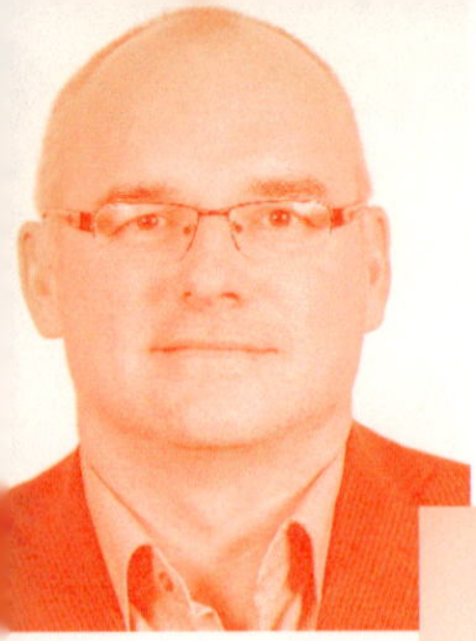
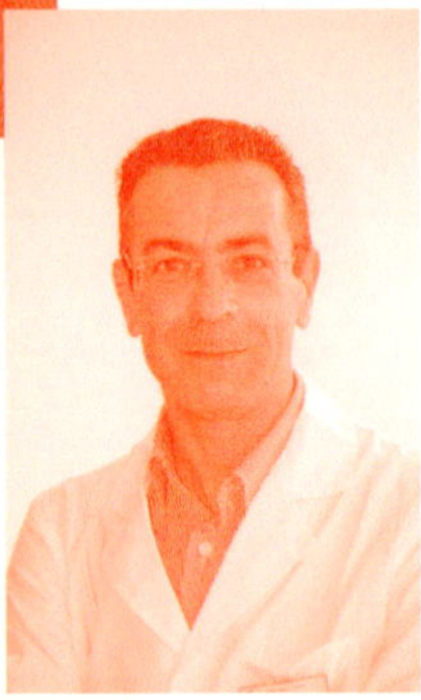
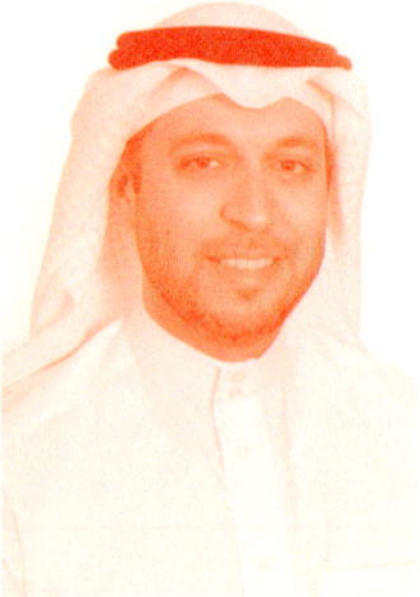
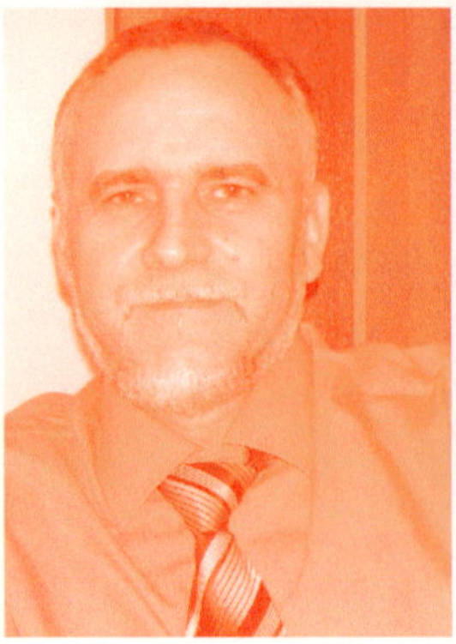
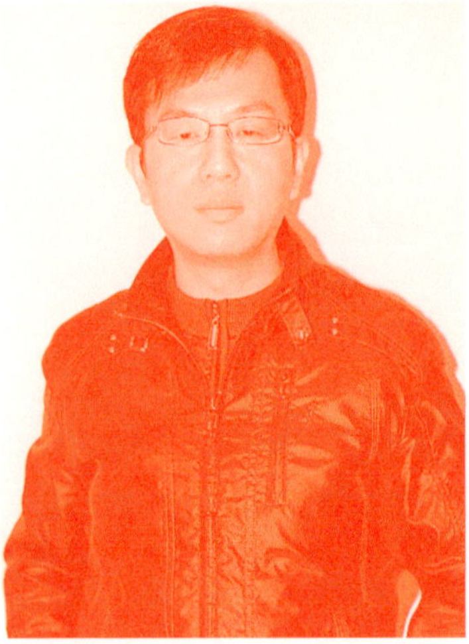
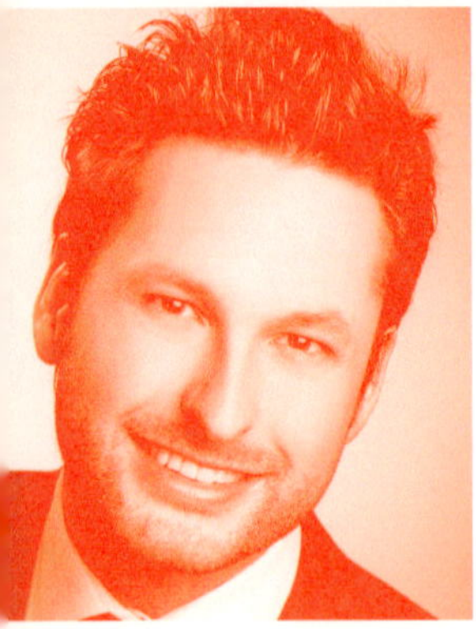
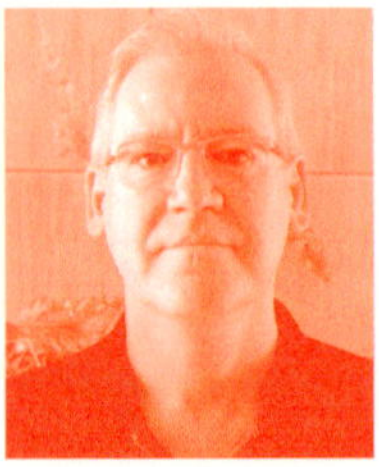

IntechOpen

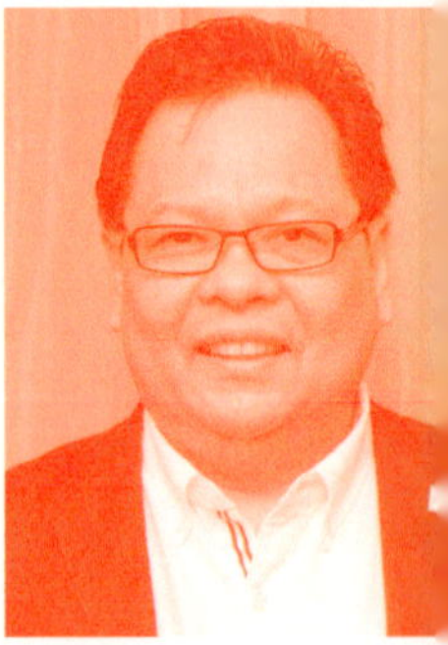
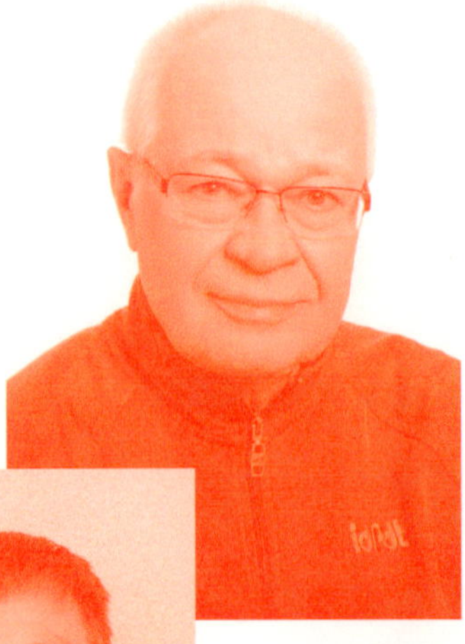
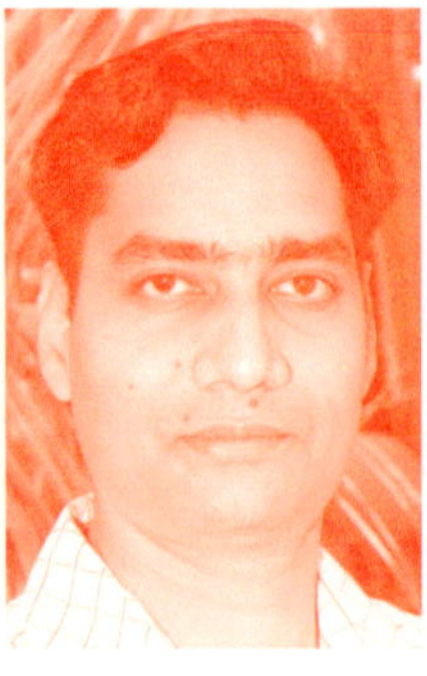
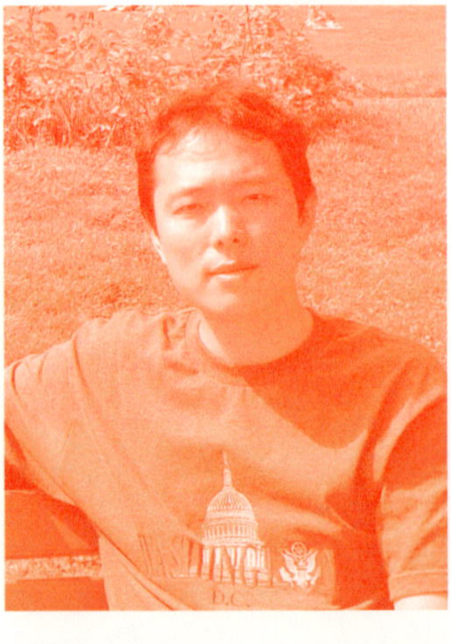
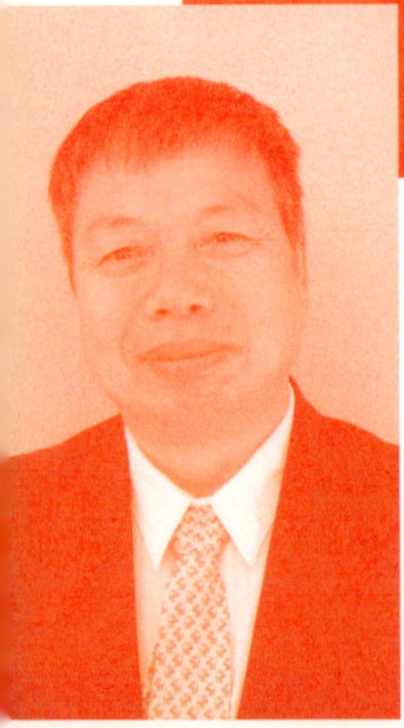
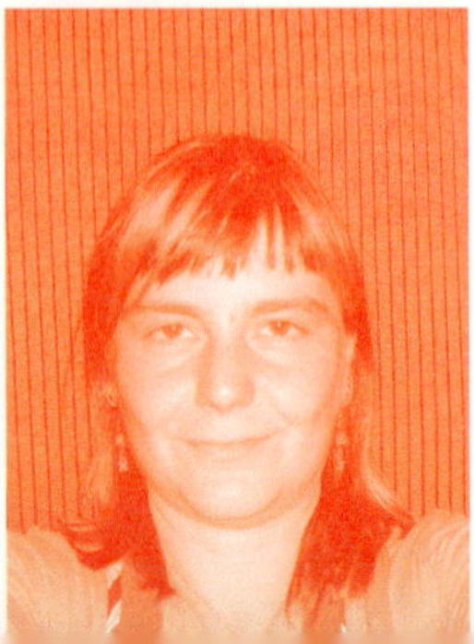

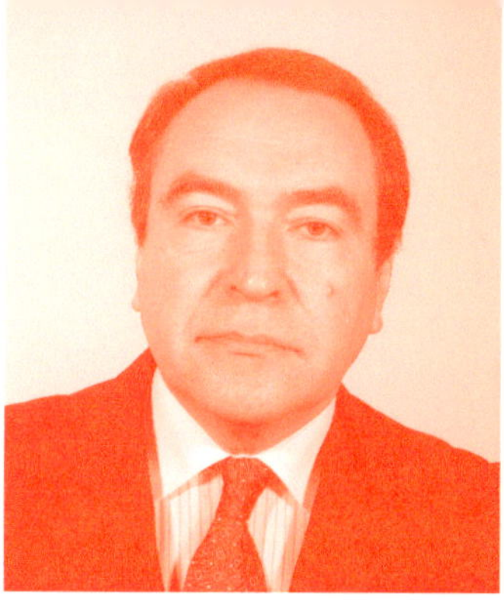
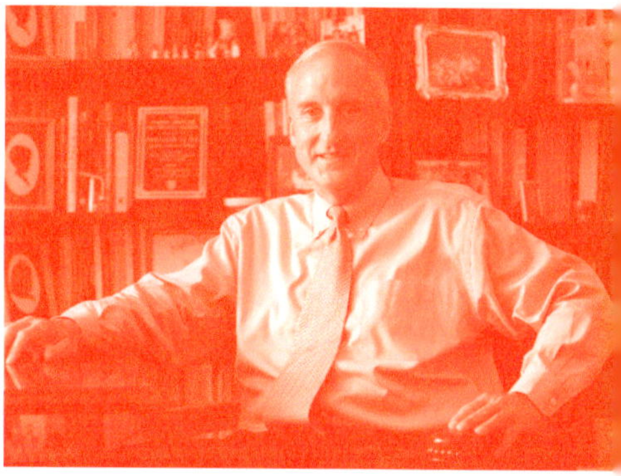
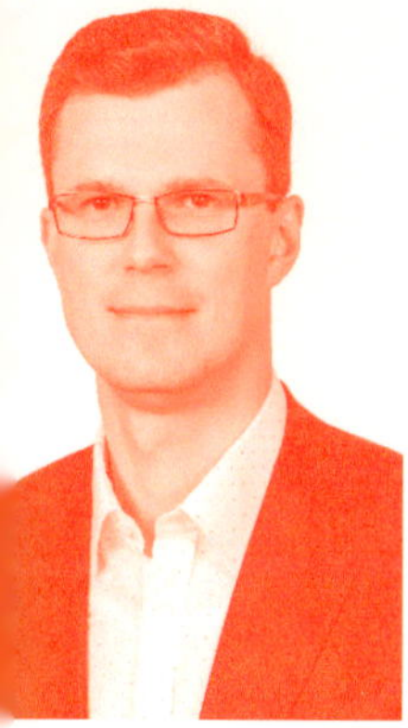
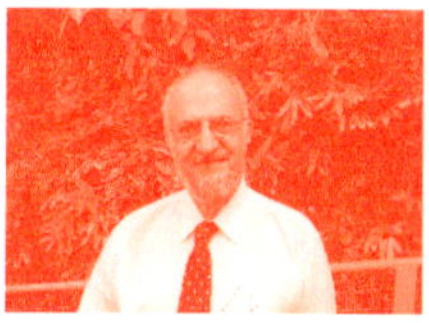
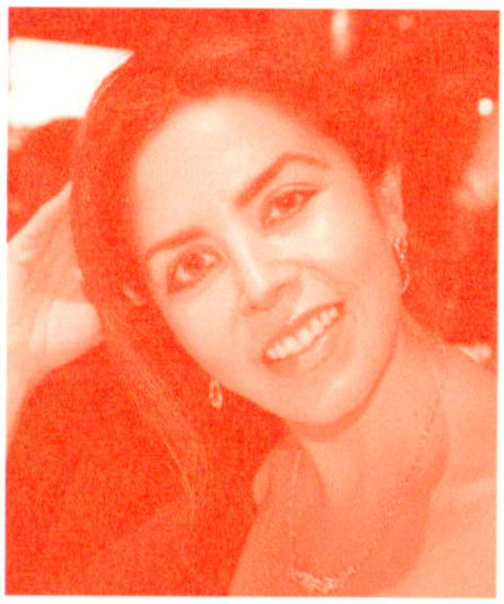

Supporting open minds since 2005

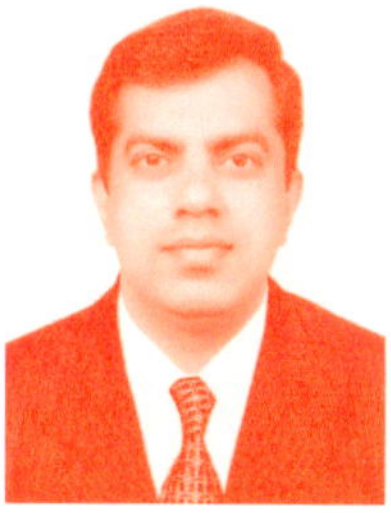
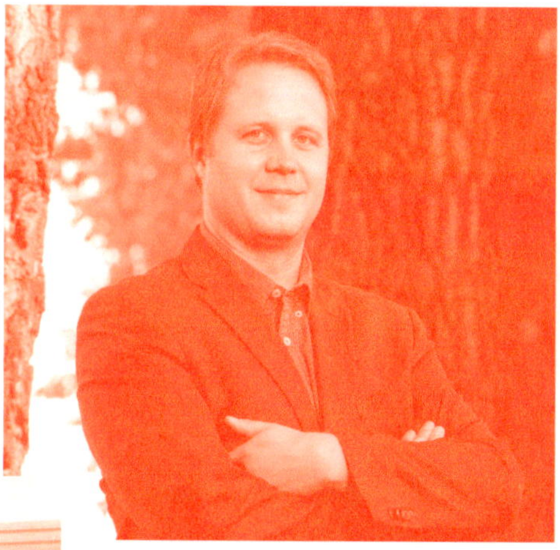
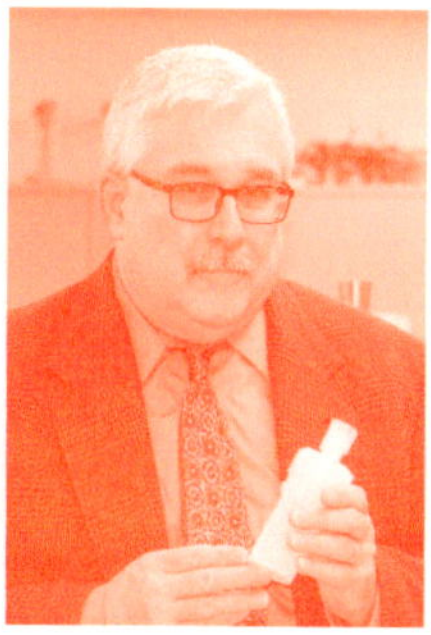
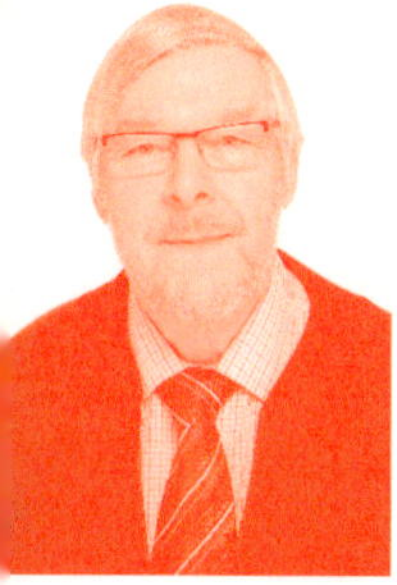
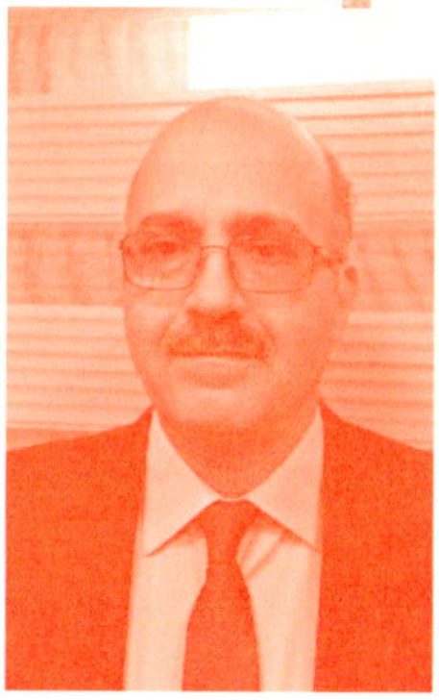
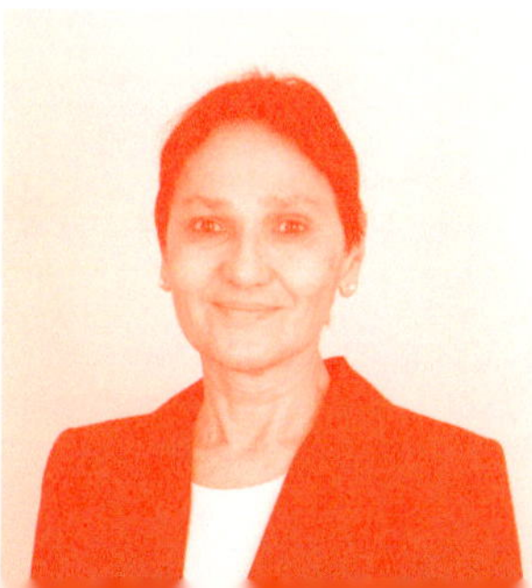
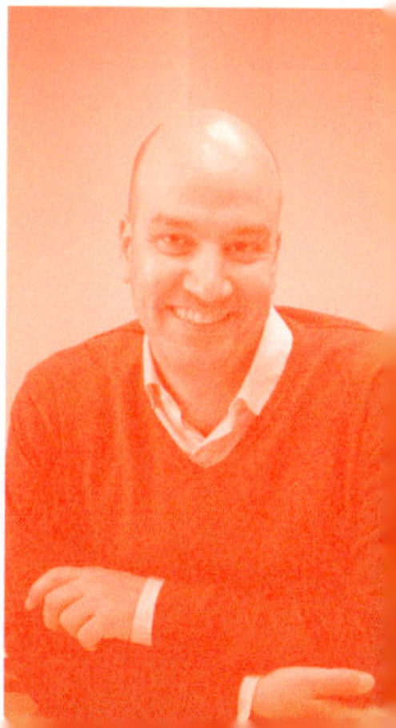

Infant Feeding - Breast versus Formula
http://dx.doi.org/10.5772/intechopen.87613
Edited by Isam Jaber Al-Zwaini, Zaid Rasheed Al-Ani and Walter Hurley

Contributors
Whitney Hamilton, Erdinc Bozkurt, Hayrunisa Bekis Bozkurt, Sandeep Kaur, Vandana Sharma, Mahima Choudhary, Simrat Kaur, Mandeep Kaur Panaich, Chandni Sharma, Sunita Chauhan, Parul Chadha, Santiago-Osorio Edelmiro, Edgar Ledesma-Martínez, Vanihamin Dominguez, Itzen Aguiñiga-Sánchez, Mohammad Hossein Khosravi, Bita Najafian, Jayashree Purkayastha, Burhan Başaran, Isam Jaber Al-Zwaini, Zaid Rasheed Al-Ani, Walter Hurley

First published in London, United Kingdom, 2020 by IntechOpen
IntechOpen is the global imprint of INTECHOPEN LIMITED, registered in England and Wales, registration number: 11086078, 5 Princes Gate Court, London, SW7 2QJ, United Kingdom
Printed in Croatia

British Library Cataloguing-in-Publication Data
A catalogue record for this book is available from the British Library

Additional hard and PDF copies can be obtained from orders@intechopen.com

Infant Feeding - Breast versus Formula
Edited by Isam Jaber Al-Zwaini, Zaid Rasheed Al-Ani and Walter Hurley
p. cm.
Print ISBN 978-1-83962-719-4
Online ISBN 978-1-83962-720-0
eBook (PDF) ISBN 978-1-83962-721-7

For EU product safety concerns:
IN TECH d.o.o., Prolaz Marije Krucifikse Kozulić 3, 51000 Rijeka, Croatia, info@intechopen.com or visit our website at intechopen.com.

Meet the editors

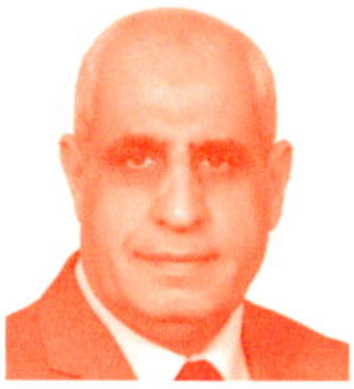

Professor Isam Jaber AL-Zwaini was born on 4 January 1963, in Baghdad, Iraq. After graduating from AL-Mustansiryia College of Medicine in 1987, he worked as a house officer in different hospitals in Baghdad for 15 months, followed by military services for 3 years. He started his pediatric study in 1991 and gained the Fellowship of Iraqi Commission for Medical Specializations in 1996. He worked as a lecturer in the Department of Pediatrics, AL-Anbar Medical College, from 1996 to 2001 when he obtained the title of Assistant Professor. In 2005, he began working in the Department of Pediatrics at AL-Kindy Medical College, University of Baghdad and obtained the title of Professor in 2008. He became an associate member of the Royal College of Pediatrics and Child Health, UK, in 2007. He served as head of the pediatric department at AL-Anbar and AL-Kindy Medical Colleges for many years. He has published more than thirty scientific papers in different pediatric fields and has a special interest in pediatric hematology, neurology, and nutrition

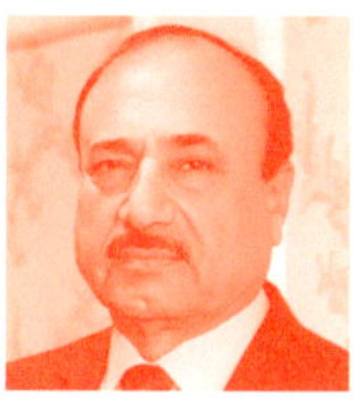

Zaid Rasheed Al-Ani obtained his Bachelor of Medicine from Basrah University in 1978, and a specialty from the Arabic Board in Pediatrics (CABP) at Baghdad University in 1992. He is currently a Professor of Pediatrics. He was on the senior pediatrics teaching staff at College of Medicine, Anbar University, where he taught and trained both undergraduate and graduate pediatrics students in nutrition, immunization, and gastroenterology. In 1992, he worked as a senior consultant pediatrician at Al-Ramadi MCH Teaching Hospital. In 2010 he served as the director and project designer of the "Western Iraqi Center for Congenital Anomalies Registry and Surveillance" in Al-Ramadi city. He is a member of several scientific discussion committees for theses of DCH, CABP, and PhD candidates. He has published more than thirteen papers in reputed journals, attended several international and local medical conferences, and is an editor and reviewer for different international journals.

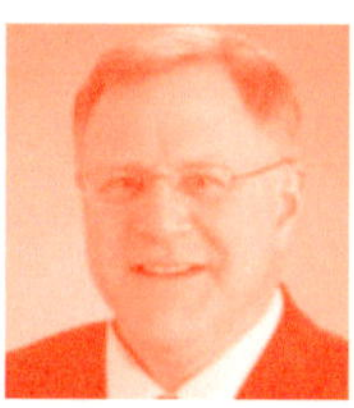

Walter L. Hurley is Professor Emeritus in the Department of Animal Sciences at the University of Illinois in Urbana, Illinois, USA. His research focuses on a broad range of topics related to the biology of lactation. His studies examine aspects of comparative milk composition, immunoglobulin transport through colostrum, lactation physiology, and mammary gland development, function, and involution in cattle and swine. He has been the recipient of a number of recognitions for his teaching, and has shared his experience and knowledge of the concepts of teaching and learning with many national and international audiences. His online, open-access Lactation Biology course (Coursera, Lactation Biology) includes more than 120 short videos, offering learners fundamental information about the biology of lactation.

Contents

Preface

Feeding during the first two years of life is very important for the nutrition and growth of an infant. The World Health Organization (WHO) ranks feeding as one of the most effective interventions for improving a child's health. It has a great effect on early morbidity and mortality and a long-term effect on the health and future of individuals and the public. Breastfeeding, formula feeding, and complementary food introduction constitute the main parts of feeding during infancy. Breastfeeding, especially when done exclusively for the first six months, has many benefits for the infant, mother, and the public in general. Formula feeding, although associated with disadvantages and problems, can be life saving for infants who need it. Introduction of complementary food at the proper time is important to meet growth requirements and prevent common nutritional problems. This book covers infant feeding and nutrition over eight chapters organized into five sections.

The first chapter is an introductory chapter written by the editors that discusses the impact of the first 1000 days of nutrition on child health and development. The concept of the first 1000 days refers to the period from conception through the age of 2 years. This period is crucial for the growth and development of fetus and child and the child's long-term health outcomes. Many factors influence this period including maternal health, breast and complementary feeding, and socioeconomic factors. Biological and metabolic development may be permanently affected by nutritional interventions, leading to adaptive pathophysiological alteration later in childhood and/or adulthood, such as the development of non-communicable disease like diabetes mellitus, cardiovascular and chronic respiratory diseases, cancers, and neurodegenerative disorders, as well as obesity. In other words, children and adult health risks may be programmed by nutritional status during this period. As such, this chapter concentrates on the effects of the first 1000 days of nutrition on the development of obesity, respiratory diseases, and the brain, as well as the role of probiotics and epigenetics.

The second chapter by Dr. Jayashree Purkayastha discusses the basic concepts of breastfeeding in normal newborns. Breastfeeding is complete nutrition for the baby and beneficial to both baby and mother. Mothers should be prepared for breastfeeding and motivated antenatally. Breastfeeding should be initiated within one hour of normal delivery and four hours of cesarean section. Colostrum is secreted within the first two days of life and is highly immunogenic to the baby. Mature milk comes by day 10 of life. Foremilk is rich in protein and vitamins and hindmilk is rich in fat. Proper technique should be followed for successful breastfeeding. Reflexes in the mother while breastfeeding are prolactin and oxytocin reflexes and reflexes in the baby are rooting, sucking, and swallowing. In the case of early discharge from the hospital, adequacy of breastfeeding should be checked at three to five days of life. Breastfeeding develops bonding between the baby and the mother, as well as promotes infant brain growth. Human milk is suitable for the baby and contains less protein and minerals than cow's milk. It also has less solute load, which is better for the immature kidneys of a baby. Breastfeeding should be performed on demand for a minimum of eight times per day. Common feeding problems in the mother are flat or inverted nipples, sore nipples, engorgement of breasts, and mastitis. Breastfeeding can be continued in case of minor febrile illness in the mother if the illness is not infectious to the baby. Otherwise, expressed breast milk should be given if the mother is unable to breastfeed.

In the third chapter, Dr. Whitney N. Hamilton reviews the factors that influence the maternal decision of which method to feed her baby. He provides an overview of the dynamic interplay between individual, interpersonal, community, and societal factors, such as policies that impact breastfeeding rates and more specifically the health of infants. The decision to formula feed or breastfeed a child typically begins with an established prenatal intention. The chapter examines the multiple dimensions influencing maternal decision-making including individual maternal characteristics, organizational factors, hospital/provider recommendations, and systematic/policy factors. It also examines the impact of infant feeding practices on early infant and childhood health outcomes. Research has demonstrated the benefits of breastfeeding on infants and early childhood, which include but are not limited to protection against common illnesses and infections, improved IQ, and even increased school attendance. Moreover, the World Health Assembly global nutrition objectives focus on encouraging breastfeeding support across all sectors in addition to implementing tailored community-based approaches, limiting the excessive marketing of infant formula, and enforcing supportive breastfeeding legislation.

In the fourth chapter, Dr. Bozkurt Erdinc discusses the relationship between ocular morbidity and infant nutrition. The nutrition of the constantly growing and developing infant even after birth has an undeniable contribution to the development of eyes, which can be considered extensions of the brain. Therefore, the elucidation of these physiological developments is valuable in terms of preventing pathological conditions. During the first six months of an infant's life, nutrition is provided through breast milk or infant formula, and after the sixth month, there is a transition to additional food. Breast milk is considered a "miracle food," with a growing body of research being undertaken to investigate its relationship with orbital diseases and indicating that breast milk reduces ocular morbidity. Breast milk is an accessible, economical, and important nutrition source for eye development and infant health. Developments in recent years have resulted in the content of formula being closer to that of breast milk, which can positively affect the neurovisional development of babies that cannot be fed with breast milk.

The fifth chapter, by E. Ledesma Martinez, is dedicated to caseins as a regulator of hematopoiesis. The main physiological role of casein, the main protein component in milk, is to be a source of amino acids that are required for the growth of the neonate; therefore, casein is considered a highly nutritious protein. Over time, it has been revealed that casein is a protein whose physiological importance reaches levels far superior to the food field, having a wide array of biological activities including antimicrobial activities, facilitating the absorption of nutrients, and acting as a growth factor and immune stimulant. The authors analyze how caseins can exert numerous hematopoietic and immunomodulatory actions and their role in granulopoiesis, monocytopoiesis, and lymphopoiesis from the early stages of postnatal development seemingly throughout life. They explore whether casein could be useful to fight pathogens resistant to antibiotics, inducing a strong immune response in immunosuppressed patients, or even be a prophylactic strategy to prevent infections.

Sandeep Kaur et al., in the sixth chapter, highlight the prophylactic and therapeutic role of human breast milk proteins and bioactive peptides against neonatal bacterial Infections. Breast milk represents nature's best mechanism to provide complete nourishment and protection to the newborn. Breastfeeding plays an important role in not only providing abundant nutrients to the infant but also acts as a storehouse of an array of bioactive factors including antimicrobial proteins and antimicrobial peptides (AMPs). These peptides help in conferring early protection and thus lowering the incidence of developing various infections such as diarrheal infections, respiratory infections, pneumonia, neonatal sepsis, enterocolitis, and others. These antimicrobial peptides also possess the property of immune modulation activating the immune cells to fight against invading pathogens and thus boosting the innate immune system. Among the bioactive peptides, endogenous peptides present in breast milk produced after cleavage by proteases have opened a new window of research focusing on studying their unique mechanisms of action. This may help in incorporating these useful peptides in formula milk for meeting special needs where breastfeeding is not possible. These properties confer human breastfeeding as an important intervention in preventing as well as treating many diseases and decreasing the rate of early child deaths. This chapter gives a deep insight into the various AMPs and the newly reported endogenous peptides present in human breast milk with emphasis on the levels and activity of AMPs in preterm milk. Also, the chapter highlights the antibacterial mechanism as well as immune modulating pathways adopted by these bioactive peptides and elucidates their protective and therapeutic role towards various clinically relevant neonatal bacterial pathogens (*Escherichia coli*, *Staphylococcal aureus*, *Streptococcus pyogenes*, *S. agalactiae*, *S. pneumoniae*, coagulase negative staphylococci (CoNS), *Klebsiella pneumoniae*, *Pseudomons aeruginosa*, etc.) with special emphasis on the infections caused by resistant bacterial strains in hospital settings (neonatal wards).

In the seventh chapter, Dr. Bita Najafian and Mohammad Hossein Khosravi review the subject of breastfeeding and gut microbiota. Human breast milk is not only a source of nutrition for infants but also contains a variety of biologically active components and bacterial species. These molecules and bacteria guide both intestinal microbiota and the infantile immune system. Recently published studies have found several vital roles for gut microbiota including effects on the individual's personality, decreased predisposition to the diseases, and a variety of other health-related consequences such as possible therapeutic or preventative effects.

The last chapter, by Dr. Burhan Başaran, discusses childhood foods and Infant formula exposure to thermal processing contaminants of furan, chloropropanols, and acrylamide by food processing. In this chapter, the author evaluates the exposure of thermal processing contaminants such as furan, chloropropanols and acrylamide from infant formulas. These compounds are produced in foods naturally as a result of thermal processing and accepted as potentially carcinogenic for humans by the International Agency for Research on Cancer. They exist at varying levels in several types of foods including infant formulas and their consumption leads to exposure. In this sense, it is apparent that humans face hidden danger through dietary exposure throughout their lives. Infants are exposed to the greatest levels of these substances due to the fact that they have low body weight and consume infant formulas in their diets as alternative nutrition.

I hope this book will shed light on some of the interesting aspects of infant feeding and nutrition. I would like to thank all authors who contributed chapters for their patience and cooperation throughout the publication of this book. I would also like to give great thanks and gratitude to the staff at IntechOpen, especially Ms. Dolores Kuzelj who offered me great help throughout the process.

Isam Jaber AL-Zwaini
Professor,
Department of Pediatrics,
AL-Kindy Medical College,
University of Baghdad,
Baghdad, Iraq

Zaid Rasheed Al-Ani
University of Anbar,
Ramadi, Iraq

Walter L. Hurley
University of Illinois,
Champaign, IL, United States of America

Section 1

Introduction

Chapter 1

Introductory Chapter: Impact of First 1000 Days Nutrition on Child Development and General Health

Isam Jaber AL-Zwaini, Zaid Rasheed AL-Ani and Walter Hurley

1. Introduction

The concept of the first 1000 days refers to the period from conception through the age of 2 years. This period is very crucial for the growth and development of the fetus and child and its long-term health outcomes. Many factors influence this period, including maternal health, breast and complementary feeding, and socioeconomic factors. Biological and metabolic development might be affected permanently by nutritional interventions, leading to adaptive pathophysiological alteration later in childhood and/or adulthood, such as noncommunicable diseases like diabetes mellitus, cardiovascular and chronic respiratory diseases, cancers and neurodegenerative disorders [1], as well as obesity and its adverse consequences [2]. In other words, children's and adults' health risks may be programmed by the nutritional status during this period. The first scientist who raised the theory of the possible effect of inherited genes and environmental factors during this critical period as an origin for the adult disease was Professor David Barker during the 1980s of the last century [3]. Barker affirmed, "Much of human development is completed during the first 1000 days after conception." His theory was later evolved in the Developmental Origin of Health and Disease (DOHaD) theory [4].

This introductory chapter aims to discuss the effects of nutrition, during pregnancy through the age of 2 years, on the health and development of the child and adult and the potential underlying mechanisms.

2. First 1000 days and overweight and/or obesity

Overweight and obesity are defined as an abnormal or excessive accumulation of fat that may impair health. It is a very common problem worldwide, and according to WHO an estimated 38.2 million children under the age of 5 were overweight or obese in 2019 and 340 million children and adolescents aged 5–19 were overweight or obese in 2016 [5]. Obese children are more likely to become obese adults, and in 2016, more than 1.9 billion adults aged 18 years and older were overweight and of these 650 million adults were obese. The problem is increasing and the worldwide prevalence of obesity nearly tripled between 1975 and 2016 [5]. There is increasing evidence that the origins of obesity are within the first 1000 days of life [6]. Prevention of childhood obesity is a public health priority and as it the source for adult obesity, early intervention is recommended. Effective and affordable preventive strategies that are embedded in the existing health system are needed.

These strategies should start early in life, should not be resource intensive, and can be maintained for the long term [7–10].

Risk factors' list for childhood obesity is wide, and antecedents are multifactorial, including genetic/epigenetic, social, biological, environmental, dietary, and behavioral influences. Among these, the most important modifiable risk factors during pregnancy and early childhood are maternal overweight/obesity, gestational weight gain, feeding practice during the first 2 years of life, in addition to maternal general health and smoking during pregnancy, physical activity, and sleep duration [6].

Although the fetal origin of the disease is an old theory dating back to about 40 years ago [3], focusing on its role in the prevention of childhood overweight/ obesity is recent. Aspects of nutritional programming are variable, and some aspects may result in a modification in organs or endocrine structures and their function, resulting in irreversible lifelong consequences, and other aspects can be corrected with repeated learned exposure as in early flavor programming for later acceptance of taste/flavor [6]. Childhood obesity is a multifactorial problem. Both acquired and environmental factors can induce effects on genetic expression, and with appropriate interventions, some of the epigenetic changes can be reversed or modified [11]. Several of these modifiable factors have been identified and well studied at the individual level. The most important are maternal feeding behavior during pregnancy and feeding practice behavior during the first 2 years of life. Generally, these factors can be categorized as food and diet behavior (maternal BMI and the rate of increase weight during pregnancy, breastfeeding, age of introduction of complementary feeding, fruit and vegetable intake, sweetened beverage consumption, and the rate of infant weight gain) or feeding and associated lifestyle behavior (maternal smoking, maternal diabetes mellitus and gestational diabetes, sleep duration or screen watching time, use of a pacifier, physical activity, parental inattention to child hunger and satiety, and the parental use of rewarding, controlling, and restrictive feeding practice behavior) [12–14].

A good example of how maternal diet affects the nutritional and metabolic programming of infants as well as his food preference is flavor programming, in which shaping infant food preferences is rooted to fetus exposure via amniotic fluid, and after the development of taste bud, it is from maternal diet preference during pregnancy. As such, the infant shows preference to carrot-flavored cereal in his complementary food when his mother consumed carrot-flavored water during the latter part of pregnancy [15].

Prevention of childhood obesity is also related to infant feeding during the first 2 years of life. Healthy growth of infants requires breastfeeding started as early as possible after birth and the introduction of nutritious complementary food at an appropriate time. Weight gain during the first year of life is one of the best predictors for later obesity [16]. When compared with formula feed counterparts, infants on breastfeeding have a lower percentage of body fat accumulation and in turn lower weight gain and risk for obesity [17]. Three meta-analyses of observational studies found that the obesity risk at school age was reduced by 15–25% with early breastfeeding compared with formula feeding. Additionally, 4% lower obesity prevalence at a later age for each additional month of breastfeeding had been reported [18].

There is no consistent evidence that the introduction of complementary feeding before the age of 4 months is associated with higher later risk for obesity when compared with the introduction of infant complementary feeding between 4 and 6 months or at 6 months age. A study involving a systematic review of the literature investigating the relationship between the introduction of complementary feeding time and overweight or obesity during childhood concludes that the risk of childhood overweight and obesity has no clear association with the timing of the introduction of complementary foods, although some evidence suggests that very early introduction (at or before 4 months), rather than at 4–6 months or more than 6 months, may increase the risk of childhood overweight [19].

Complementary diet quantity and quality, and in turn energy intake, may also play a role in the acquisition of subsequent childhood obesity. A large study that followed 881 infants in the United Kingdom shows that a higher prevalence of greater weight gain between birth and 1–3 years of age can be predicted in infants who were provided with solid foods at the age of 4 months [20].

Higher dietary protein intake during infancy, in particular from infant formula, had been found to be associated with a higher risk of obesity during the first 6 years of life [18, 21]. One explanation is given through early protein hypothesis, which describes the increasing level of insulin and insulin-like growth factor-1 as a result of high protein intake in early life, resulting in increased fat deposition and weight gain [18]. Apart from sweetened beverage intake, total carbohydrate intake during complementary feeding seems not to be associated with a higher risk of later childhood obesity [22]. Most of the studies about the role of fat intake during infancy in the development of childhood obesity failed to show a positive relationship. Although, one large study from China concludes that fat intake as fish liver oil is associated with a higher risk of childhood overweight [23, 24].

Measures to decrease the risk of obesity through the behavioral changes and nutritional education are found to be most effective during early life. Furthermore, human biology is the most pliable and amenable to changes during this period [25, 26].

3. First 1000 days nutrition and respiratory diseases

Susceptibility to the development of respiratory disease and its progression is affected by nutrition and feeding during the first 1000 days through epigenetic mechanisms [27]. Additionally, nutrition might affect the development of microbiota, which in turn can impress inflammatory, allergic, and immune mechanisms, rendering some individuals more susceptible to the various respiratory diseases of various mechanisms [28]. A study by Mayor et al. in 2015 shows that placental developmental and fetal growth is affected by poor maternal nutrition, resulting in increased susceptibility to noncommunicable diseases. This study in particular revealed that a high maternal fat diet intake before and during pregnancy increased glucose and insulin levels, leading to placental inflammation resulting in placental insufficiency, intrauterine growth restriction, and alteration of fetal lung development [29]. Fetal lung maturation impairment predisposes the neonate to an increased risk of respiratory distress syndrome at birth and chronic lung disease later on [30]. Furthermore, intake of diets rich in vegetables and fruit in the first and second trimesters is associated with a lower risk for allergic respiratory diseases such as allergic rhinitis and asthma in contrast with a diet rich in vegetable oil, margarine, and processed food [31]. This is very important when we compare Western diet (rich in oil, fast food, and processed food) to the Mediterranean diet (rich in fruit and vegetable, olive oil, fish, cereals, and other fiber diets) as a maternal dietary risk factor for the development of respiratory diseases. The adherence to the Mediterranean diet has been found to be associated with the normalization trend of gut microbiota, making it a good preventive choice for allergic diseases [32]. Some studies show that maternal supplementation with fish source Omega-3 polyunsaturated long-chain fatty acids during pregnancy is associated with a lower risk of allergic sensitization like allergic rhinitis, asthma, and atopic dermatitis [31, 33, 34]. Additionally, maternal supplementation during pregnancy with micronutrients as Vitamin D and E and zinc is associated with a lower risk for childhood wheezes [35].

The short- and long-term benefits of breastfeeding are beyond doubt. Breastfeeding reduces childhood morbidity and mortality from infectious diseases, including respiratory, because it contains secretory IgA antibodies, anti-inflammatory cytokines, galacto-oligosaccharides, and lactoferrin [36]. The American Academy of Pediatrics reported, in 2012, a 72% reduction of risk of first-year hospitalization in exclusively breastfed infants for the first 4 months of life. Additionally, the severity of RSV bronchiolitis was reduced by 74% when compared with infants who are never or only partially breastfed [37]. WHO, on the other hand, reports that human milk can reduce the rate of hospital admission, severity, and mortality of lower respiratory tract infection by around 50, 30, and 60%, respectively [38].

The increasing incidence of various types of allergic diseases, including allergic rhinitis and asthma, in the last decades, is well documented all over the world, especially in developed countries. Many theories for this raise of incidence have been suggested, such as the urbanization of the population and following of the western lifestyle. Hygiene hypothesis (decreased rate of infectious burden is associated with the increased incidence of allergic disease), tobacco smoking, pollution, sedentary lifestyle, and reduced rate or absence of breastfeeding in the first months of life are thought to be important contributors [31]. In the first year of life, exposure to a wide range of food antigens is associated with a lower incidence of asthma, allergic rhinitis, and atopic dermatitis. So, the inclusion of food allergen in the first year of life might be protective against allergic diseases especially asthma [31]. Furthermore, maternal diet during pregnancy might have an impact on health even before delivery, and some interventional studies report immunomodulatory effects of specific nutrients on the neonate and a reduction of early sensitization to allergens [39, 40]. The proposed mechanisms are mainly immunological, suggesting the key role of diet in the hemostasis of the immune system, leading to oral tolerance and preventing excessive reactions to innocuous antigens which lead to allergic disease.

The role of breastfeeding in preventing allergic respiratory disease is controversial. Some studies have addressed the protective effect of breast feeding on the development of allergic diseases during childhood by facilitating the development of host immune mechanisms especially against allergic rhinitis in the first 5 years of life, while the evidence for the association between breastfeeding and wheezing and asthma was inconclusive [41, 42]. On the other hand, a protective effect of exclusive breastfeeding during the first 3 months of life against the development of asthma in children from atopic families has been demonstrated by other recent studies [29].

Many studies have investigated the role of complementary foods' introduction during infancy as a risk factor for developing allergy. Delayed introduction of solid foods has no effects on the prevalence of allergy, a result found by many studies [43, 44]. Recently, many studies investigated the protective effect of early introduction of highly allergenic foods (cow's milk, egg, fish, and peanuts) after at least 3–4 months of exclusive breastfeeding against food allergy [30]. In general, the results of these studies and many others [31, 45, 46] are inconclusive, and further studies, especially in children with a positive family history of atopy, are required to investigate the role of timing of introduction of high allergenic food in the development of atopy.

The effect of type of the diet on the susceptibility to asthma and atopy in children also has been studied. It has been found that Mediterranean type of diet (rich in fruit, vegetable, fibers, seafood, and olive oil) has a protective effect against asthma and atopy when compared to the western style of diet (rich in saturated fats, red meats and poor in fruit, vegetable, whole grain, and seafood) [33, 47].

The micronutrient also has an important protective effect against respiratory diseases. Those with a potent antioxidant activity may delay the onset, severity, and outcome of asthma. Recent studies conclude that asthma is associated with the boosted production of reactive oxygen and reactive nitrogen species (ROS and RNS) and the pathogenesis of this disease is enhanced by changes in enzymatic antioxidant activity in lung and blood. Furthermore, both ROS and RNS increase systemic oxidative stress and subsequently increase the oxidative burden due to the alteration of systemic and blood antioxidant systems, which is typical of bronchial asthma. Wherefore, improvement of antioxidant activity may represent a successful strategy for delaying the onset, decreasing the severity, and improving the outcome of asthma. The most important antioxidants in this regard are vitamin E, vitamin C, selenium, coenzyme Q10, and carotene [48]. Zinc and iron have an important role in the immune system. Zinc is thought to inhibit the viral replication or intracellular adhesion and boost immune response at mucosal surfaces and hence may have a protective effect against the upper respiratory tract infections. Iron, on the other hand, has an important role in cytokines secretion, T cell proliferation, and bactericidal activity. Iron deficiency might impair these functions [48].

Vitamins also play a role in the defense mechanisms against respiratory diseases. Vitamin A is important for the enhancement of immune function and may limit the severity of respiratory infections in children older than 5 years of age [30]. Vitamin D, on the other hand, probably affects the onset, severity, and exacerbation of asthma, respiratory tract infections, and chronic obstructive airway diseases. Many theories have been adopted to explain this effect of vitamin D, including modulating immune mechanisms [49] and its influences on fetal lung maturation and airway smooth muscle cell proliferation and differentiation per via paracrine [50]. The role of vitamin C in the prevention and treatment of common cold is well known. By its potent antioxidant proprieties, vitamin C counteracts oxidants and decreases the external attacks of bacteria, viruses, toxins, and xenobiotics in the lung and hence modulates the development of bronchial inflammation and the impairment of pulmonary function [30, 51]. Contrary to the positive effects of the above vitamins, some studies show that folic acid (commonly used as a preventive measure for neural tube defects) in high dose given after the first trimester has been associated with an increased incidence of childhood asthma and eczema [30]. This relationship has not been documented by many other studies [52, 53].

4. First 1000 days nutrition and brain development

Throughout life, the first 1000 days represent the most vulnerable period for brain development and growth. During this period, the brain grows more rapidly than any other time, and it is the period where the neuronal connection and proper cognitive functioning occurs. Nutritional needs should be met during this period to ensure proper growth and development of the brain. A lifelong deficit may result from failure to provide key nutrients during this critical period despite subsequent nutrient repletion [54].

Development of the brain started 16 days after conception, growing throughout pregnancy, and taking adult form by 7 months of gestation [55]. Protein, fat and fatty acids, zinc, iron, folate, and iodine are required for neuronal creation, myelination, and synapses formation. Inadequate intake for these nutrients and micronutrients might impair the neurodevelopmental process [56].

Nutrition during the first 2 years of life is essential for this critical period of brain development and growth. Motor functions such as posture, balance, and coordination and the child's ability to create and recall memories (hippocampal—prefrontal connection) are well known to develop during this period [57]. Breastfeeding is the idealistic food for brain growth and development during the first 2 years of life as it contains hormones, growth factors, and a variety of nutrients that are essential for this process. Deoni et al., in their cross-sectional study in 2013, conclude that infant breastfeeding is associated with improved developmental growth in late-maturing white matter association regions, and extended breastfeeding duration is associated with improved white matter structure and cognitive performance [58]. Furthermore, extreme preterm infants fed predominatingly with breast milk in the first 28 days of life show a greater deep nuclear gray matter volume, and by the age of 7 years, they had higher IQs and better scores in reading, mathematics, working memory, and motor function tests [59]. Breastfeeding provides not only the first-class nutrition necessary for the shaping of the brain but also affects the quality of the experiences and interactions they have with caregivers, which is found to be critical for both the cognitive and socio-emotional development [60].

5. First 1000 days nutrition and probiotics

The term dysbiosis refers to the microbial imbalance inside the human, especially digestive tract. In the last two decades, there was a great interest in the human microbiome. Thousands of studies were conducted to highlight its impact on health and disease. More than 500 bacteria species were found harboring the digestive tract, representing about 25 times more genes than the human genome [61, 62]. These microbes are thought to play a vital role in human health through protection against pathogenic microorganisms, metabolic functions by fermentation of indigestible carbohydrates, and modulation of the human immune system. Furthermore, recently there is important evidence to link dysbiosis with many human diseases like allergy, asthma, obesity, and inflammatory bowel diseases [63–65]. The gut of newborns will be rapidly colonized by microbes immediately after birth from exposure to the mother's microbiota, especially from the vagina and fecal material. Later on, feeding, close physical contact like hugging and kissing, and the environment will be the source of microbes. The adult pattern of gut microbiota will be established by the age of 3 years [66]. The establishment of the gut bacterial patterns is greatly influenced by the type of feeding. Breast milk is rich in complex nondigestible oligosaccharides, with more than 200 different molecules [67]. These oligosaccharides are resistant to hydrolysis by human small intestine enzymes and reach the large intestine, acting as substrates for microorganisms there, promoting the growth of specific bacteria. Nowadays, most infant formulas are supplemented with oligosaccharides, in particular fructo- and galacto-oligosaccharides, with the aim to improve the intestinal microbiota in early life [68]. Early dysbiosis that resulted from different factors like cesarean sections, prematurity, and early exposure to antibiotics might be associated with a wide spectrum of diseases like obesity, allergic disease, and autism spectrum disorders as revealed by several epidemiological studies [68, 69].

6. First 1000 days and epigenetics

Epigenetic modifications of the expression of genes occur through several mechanisms including DNA methylation, histone modifications, and posttranscriptional gene-silencing by noncoding microRNAs [1]. Modifications to the epigenetic profile by external and internal environments of the cell can have short-term and long-term effects on gene expression [70–72]. A range of environmental stressors have epigenetic effects that are associated with diseases [70]. Some of these stressors include tobacco smoke-related diseases, air pollution effects on immunity and inflammatory responses, endocrine disrupting compounds, and others [73, 74].

Studies of the impact of environmental stressors on the epigenome provide insights into the mechanisms that link those stressors with the subsequent manifestations of disease. Such studies are especially important in establishing a full understanding of the linkage between stressor-induced modifications of the epigenome during the initial 1000 days and maternal and neonatal nutrition. At this time, most human studies have been aimed at characterizing the degree of association between epigenetic modifications and environmental stressors. Many of these studies use methodologies that characterize changes in global DNA methylation patterns or methylation of a limited subset of specific genes of interest in cord blood or maternal or neonatal peripheral blood samples. The methylation patterns are then used as biomarkers to correlate with the developmental abnormalities and disease status. A few examples are summarized here.

Maternal folate nutrition during pregnancy has been implicated in several birth defects [75]. The mechanisms that underlie DNA methylation are dependent on dietary folate and one-carbon metabolism [76]. Methylation profiles of a number of genes, including some not normally associated with folate biology, have a significant association with the maternal plasma folate during pregnancy [77]. Maternal serum folate concentrations are associated with DNA methylation patterns of seven genomic regions observed in the neonatal cord blood, especially in a region upstream of a regulator of DNA methylation during development [78]. Methylation patterns of insulin-like growth factor-2 (*IGF2*) in children are associated with the maternal periconceptional supplementation of folic acid [79]. Others have observed that the methylation patterns of *IGF2* promoter regions are not associated with the folate concentrations in maternal blood or cord blood [80]. On the other hand, the latter study did report an association between the serum levels of vitamin B12 in maternal blood and methylation patterns in one of the *IGF2* promoters. Vitamin D supplementation of pregnant and lactating women also has been associated with differential epigenome-wide DNA methylation patterns in their breastfed infants [81]. Specific effects of folate and other nutrients on epigenetic alterations in the fetus or newborn continue to be the areas of active investigation.

Toxic metal (arsenic, mercury, cadmium, and lead) exposure during pregnancy is associated with epigenomic changes in the offspring [82, 83]. Similarly, epigenomic changes in the offspring have been found associated with the exposure to endocrine disruptors, such as bisphenol-a, dichlorodiphenyltrichloroethane, polybrominated diphenyl ethers, polychlorinated biphenyls, and phthalates [83]. The relationship between these types of observed associations of epigenetic changes and environmental stressors during pregnancy and early life and their relationship with the known effects of those stressors and childhood and adult health remain to be understood.

Prenatal exposure to famine is associated with less methylation of the insulin-like growth factor-2 (*IGF2*) gene observed in adults six decades later [84]. That study underscores the potential for early life environmental stressors to cause long-term epigenetic modifications. Prenatal exposure to other environmental stressors on the mother, such as smoking, asthma, immune stress during pregnancy, and obesity, are associated with differences in the DNA methylation patterns of peripheral blood cells when comparing children who develop asthma with those who do not develop the condition [85].

Author details

Isam Jaber AL-Zwaini[1*], Zaid Rasheed AL-Ani[2] and Walter Hurley[3]

1 Department of Pediatrics, AL-Kindy College of Medicine, Baghdad University, Baghdad, Iraq

2 Department of Pediatrics, AL-Anbar College of Medicine, AL-Anbar University, AL-Anbar, Iraq

3 Department of Animal Science, University of Illinois at Urbana-Champaign, USA

*Address all correspondence to: isamjaber@kmc.uobaghdad.edu.iq

References

[1] Agosti M, Tandoi F, Morlacchi L. Angela Bossi. Nutritional and metabolic programming during the first thousand days of life. La Pediatria Medica e Chirurgica. 2017;**39**:157. DOI: 10.4081/pmc.2017.15

[2] Blake-Lamb TL, Locks LM, Perkins ME, Woo Baidal JA, Cheng ER, Taveras EM. Interventions for childhood obesity in the first 1,000 days: A systematic review. American Journal of Preventive Medicine. 2016;**50**(6):780-789. DOI: 10.1016/j.amepre.2015.11.010. Epub 6 Feb 22

[3] Barker DJ. The fetal and infant origins of adult disease. BMJ. 1990;**301**:1111

[4] Wadhwa PD, Buss C, Entringer S, Swanson JM. Developmental origins of health and disease: Brief history of the approach and current focus on epigenetic mechanisms. Seminars in Reproductive Medicine. WHO Fact Sheet. 2009;**27**(5):358-368. DOI: 10.1055/s-0029-1237424. Available from: https://www.who.int/news-room/fact sheets/detail/obesity-and-overweight

[5] WHO Fact Sheet. Available from: https://www.who.int/news-room/fact sheets/detail/obesity-and-overweight

[6] Black RE, Makrides M, Ong KK, editors. Complementary feeding: Building the foundations for a healthy life. In: Nestlé Nutr Inst Workshop Ser. Vol. 87. Basel: Nestec Ltd., Vevey/S. Karger AG; 2017. pp. 183-196. DOI: 10.1159/000448966

[7] Wake M. The failure of anti-obesity programmes in schools. BMJ. 2018;**360**:k507

[8] Blake-Lamb TL, Locks LM, Perkins ME, et al. Interventions for childhood obesity in the first 1,000 days a systematic review. American Journal of Preventive Medicine. 2016;**50**(6):780-789

[9] World Health Organization. Consideration of the evidence on childhood obesity for the commission on ending childhood obesity. In: Report of the ad hoc Working Group on Science and Evidence for Ending Childhood Obesity. Geneva, Switzerland: World Health Organization; 2016

[10] Waters E, de Silva-Sanigorski A, Hall BJ, et al. Interventions for preventing obesity in children. Cochrane Database of Systematic Reviews. 2011;**12**:CD001871

[11] World Health Organization. Interim Report of the Commission on Ending Childhood Obesity. Geneva: WHO; 2015

[12] Dattilo AM, Birch L, Krebs NF, et al. Need for early interventions in the prevention of pediatric overweight: A review and upcoming directions. Journal of Obesity. 2012;**2012**:123023

[13] Weng SF, Redsell SA, Swift JA, et al. Systematic review and meta-analyses of risk factors for childhood overweight identifiable during infancy. Archives of Disease in Childhood. 2012;**97**:1019-1026

[14] Woo Baidal JA, Locks LM, Cheng ER, Blake-Lamb TL, Perkins ME, Taveras EM. Risk factors for childhood obesity in the first 1000 days: A Systematic Review. American Journal of Preventive Medicine. 2016;**50**(6):761-779. DOI: S0749-3797(15)00752-7

[15] Shin D, Lee KW, Song WO. Pre-pregnancy weight status is associated with diet quality and nutritional biomarkers during pregnancy. Nutrients. 2016;**8**:162

[16] Ong KK, Loos RJ. Rapid infancy weight gain and subsequent obesity:

Systematic reviews and hopeful suggestions. Acta Paediatrica. 2006;**95**:904-908

[17] Dewey KG. Growth characteristics of breastfed compared to formula-fed infants. Biology of the Neonate. 1998;**74**:94-105

[18] Koletzko B, von Kries R, Closa R, et al. Can infant feeding choices modulate later obesity risk? The American Journal of Clinical Nutrition. 2009;**89**:1502S-1508S

[19] Pearce J, Taylor MA, Langley-Evans SC. Timing of the introduction of complementary feeding and risk of childhood obesity: A systematic review. International Journal of Obesity. 2013;**37**(10):1295-1306. DOI: 10.1038/ijo.2013.99

[20] Ong KK, Emmett PM, Noble S, et al. Dietary energy intake at the age of 4 months predicts postnatal weight gain and childhood body mass index. Pediatrics. 2006;**117**:e503-e508

[21] Weber M, Grote V, Closa-Monasterolo R, et al. Lower protein content in infant formula reduces BMI and obesity risk at school age: Follow-up of a randomized trial. The American Journal of Clinical Nutrition. 2014;**99**:1041-1051

[22] Pan L, Li R, Park S, et al. A longitudinal analysis of sugar-sweetened beverage intake in infancy and obesity at 6 years. Pediatrics. 2014;**134**(suppl 1):S29-S35

[23] Butte NF, Fox MK, Briefel RR, et al. Nutrient intakes of US infants, toddlers, and preschoolers meet or exceed dietary reference intakes. Journal of the American Dietetic Association. 2010;**110**:S27-S37

[24] Zheng JS, Liu H, Zhao YM, et al. Complementary feeding and childhood adiposity in preschool-aged children in a large Chinese cohort. The Journal of Pediatrics. 2015;**166**:326-331

[25] Contento IR. Nutrition education: Linking research, theory, and practice. Asia Pacific Journal of Clinical Nutrition. 2008;**17**(Suppl 1):176-179

[26] World Health Organization. Health Education: Theoretical Concepts, Effective Strategies and Core Competencies: A Foundation Document to Guide Capacity Development of Health Educators. Geneva: WHO; 2012

[27] Barker DJP. Developmental origins of chronic disease. Public Health. 2012;**126**:185-189

[28] Di Mauro A, Neu J, Riezzo G, Raimondi F, Martinelli D, Francavilla R, et al. Gastrointestinal function development and microbiota. Italian Journal of Pediatrics. 2013;**39**:15

[29] Mayor RS, Finch KE, Zehr J, Morselli E, Neinast MD, Frank AP, et al. Maternal high-fat diet is associated with impaired fetal lung development. American Journal of Physiology. Lung Cellular and Molecular Physiology. 2015;**309**:360-368

[30] Verducia E, Martellib A, Minielloc VL, et al. Nutrition in the first 1000 days and respiratory health: A descriptive review of the last five years' literature. Allergol Immunopathol (Madr). 2017;**45**(4):405-413

[31] Julia V, Macia L, Dombrowicz D. The impact of diet on asthma and allergic diseases. Nature Reviews. Immunology. 2015;**15**:308-322

[32] Bifulco M. Mediterranean diet: The missing link between gut microbiota and inflammatory disease. European Journal of Clinical Nutrition. 2015;**69**:1078

[33] Berthon BS, Wood LG. Nutrition and respiratory health --- feature review. Nutrients. 2015;7:1618-1643

[34] de Silva D, Geromi M, Halken S, Host A, Panesar SS, Muraro A, et al. Primary prevention of food allergy in children and adults: Systematic review. Allergy. 2014;**69**:581-589

[35] Beckhaus AA, Garcia-Marcos L, Forno E, Pacheco-Gonzalez RM, Celedon JC, Castro-Rodriguez JA. Maternal nutrition during pregnancy and risk of asthma, wheeze, and atopic diseases during childhood: A systematic review and meta-analysis. Allergy. 2015;**70**:1588-1604

[36] Verduci E, Banderali G, Barberi S, Radaelli G, Lops A, Betti F, et al. Epigenetics effects of human breast milk. Nutrients. 2014;**6**:1711-1724

[37] American Academy of Pediatrics (AAP). Section on breastfeeding. Breastfeeding and the use of human milk. Pediatrics. 2012;**129**:e827-e841

[38] Horta BL, Victora CG. Respiratory infection. In: Short Term Effects of Breastfeeding. A Systematic Review on the Benefits of Breastfeeding on Diarrhoea and Pneumonia Mortality. World Health Organization; 2013. pp. 30-33. Available from: http://apps.who.int/iris/bitstream/10665/95585/1/9789241506120 eng.pdf?ua=1 [Accessed: 03 July 2020]

[39] Dunstan JA et al. Fish oil supplementation in pregnancy modifies neonatal allergen-specific immune responses and clinical outcomes in infants at high risk of atopy: A randomized, controlled trial. The Journal of Allergy and Clinical Immunology. 2003;**112**:1178-1184

[40] Bunyavanich S et al. Peanut, milk, and wheat intake during pregnancy is associated with reduced allergy and asthma in children. The Journal of Allergy and Clinical Immunology. 2014;**133**:1373-1382

[41] Lodge CJ, Tan DJ, Lau MX, Dai X, Tham R, Lowe AJ, et al. Breastfeeding and asthma and allergies: A systematic review and meta-analysis. Acta Paediatrica. 2015;**104**:38-53.15

[42] Cesar GV, Bahl R, Barros AJD, GVA F, Horton S, Krasevec J, et al. Breastfeeding in the 21st century: Epidemiology, mechanisms, and lifelong effect. Lancet. 2016;**387**(10017):475-490

[43] Snijders BE, Thijs C, van Ree R, van den Brandt PA. Age at first introduction of cow milk products and other food products in relation to infant atopic manifestations in the first 2 years of life: The KOALA birth cohort study. Pediatrics. 2008;**122**:e115-e122

[44] Zutavern A, Brockow I, Schaaf B, von Berg A, Diez U, Borte M, et al. Timing of solid food introduction in relation to eczema, asthma, allergic rhinitis, and food and inhalant sensitization at the age of 6 years: Results from the prospective birth cohort study LISA. Pediatrics. 2008;**121**:e44-e52

[45] Muraro A, Halken S, Arshad SH, Beyer K, Dubois AE, Du Toit G, et al. EAACI food allergy and anaphylaxis guidelines. Primary prevention of food allergy. Allergy. 2014;**69**:590-601

[46] Alessandri C, Zennaro D, Scala E, Ferrara R, Bernardi ML, Santoro M, et al. Ovomucoid (Gal d 1) specific IgE detected by microarray system predict tolerability to boiled hen's egg and an increased risk to progress to multiple environmental allergen sensitisation. Clinical and Experimental Allergy. 2012;**42**:441-450

[47] Castro-Rodriguez JA, Ramirez-Hernandez M, Padilla O, Pacheco-Gonzalez RM, Pérez-Fernández V, Garcia-Marcos L. Effect of foods and Mediterranean diet during pregnancy and first years of life on wheezing, rhinitis and dermatitis in preschoolers. Allergol Immunopathol (Madr).

2016;**44**(5):400-409. DOI: 10.1016/j.aller.2015.12.002

[48] Fabian E, Pölöskey P, Kósa L, Elmadfa I, Réthy LA. Nutritional supplements and plasma antioxidants in childhood asthma. Wiener Klinische Wochenschrift. 2013;**125**:309-315

[49] Hossein-nezhad A, Vitamin Holick MF. D for health: A global perspective. Mayo Clinic Proceedings. 2013;**88**:720-755

[50] Bantz SK, Zhu Z, Zheng T. The role of vitamin D in pediatric asthma. Annals of Pediatrics & Child Health. 2015;**3**:1032

[51] McEvoy CT, Schilling D, Clay N, Jackson K, Go MD, Spitale P, et al. Vitamin C supplementation for pregnant smoking women and pulmonary function in their newborn infants: A randomized clinical trial. Journal of the American Medical Association. 2014;**311**:2074-2082

[52] Granell R, Heron J, Lewis S, Davey Smith G, Sterne JA, Henderson J. The association between mother and child MTHFR C677T polymorphisms, dietary folate intake and childhood atopy in a population-based, longitudinal birth cohort. Clinical and Experimental Allergy. 2008;**38**:320-328

[53] Miyake Y, Sasaki S, Tanaka K, Maternal HY. B vitamin intake during pregnancy and wheeze and eczema in Japanese infants aged 16---24 months: The Osaka Maternal and child health study. Pediatric Allergy and Immunology. 2011;**22**:69-74

[54] Schwarzenberg SJ, Georgieff MK, AAP Committee on Nutrition. Advocacy for improving nutrition in the first 1000 days to support childhood development and adult health. Pediatrics. 2018;**141**(2):e20173716

[55] Couperus JW, Nelson CA. Early brain development and plasticity. In: McCartney K, Phillips D, editors. Blackwell Handbook of Early Childhood Development. Oxford, UK: Blackwell Publishing Ltd.; 2006

[56] Georgieff MK, Rao R, Fuglestad AJ. The role of nutrition in cognitive development. In: Nelson CA, Luciana M, editors. Handbook of Developmental Cognitive Neuroscience. Cambridge, MA: MIT Press; 1999. pp. 491-504

[57] Williams J, Mai CT, Isenbrug J, et al. Updated estimates of neural tube defects prevented by mandatory folic acid fortification in the United States 1995-2011. Morbidity and Mortality Weekly Report. 2015;**64**(01):1-5

[58] Deoni SC, Dean DC 3rd, Piryatinsky I, et al. Breastfeeding and early white matter development: A cross-sectional study. NeuroImage. 2013;**82**:77-86. DOI: 10.1016/j.neuroimage.2013.05.090

[59] Belfort MB, Anderson PJ, Nowak VA, et al. Breast Milk feeding, brain development, and neurocognitive outcomes: A 7-year longitudinal study in infants born at less than 30 Weeks' gestation. The Journal of Pediatrics. 2016;**177**:133-139.e1. DOI: 10.1016/j.jpeds.2016.06.045

[60] Lee H, Park H, Ha E, et al. Effect of breastfeeding duration on cognitive development in infants: 3-year follow-up study. Journal of Korean Medical Science. 2016;**31**(4):579-584. DOI: 10.3346/jkms.2016.31.4.579

[61] Qin J, Li R, Raes J, et al. A human gut microbial gene catalogue established by metagenomic sequencing. Nature. 2010;**464**:59-65

[62] Dietert RR, Dietert JM. The microbiome and sustainable healthcare. Healthcare. 2015;**3**:100-129

[63] Butel M, Waligora-Dupriet A, Wydau-Dematteis S. The developing

gut microbiota and its consequences for health. Journal of Developmental Origins of Health and Disease. 2018;**9**(6):590-597. DOI: 10.1017/S2040174418000119

[64] Fujimura KE, Slusher NA, Cabana MD, Lynch SV. Role of the gut microbiota in defining human health. Expert Review of Anti-Infective Therapy. 2010;**8**:435-454

[65] Neish AS. Microbes in gastrointestinal health and disease. Gastroenterology. 2009;**136**:65-80

[66] Yatsunenko T, Rey FE, Manary MJ, et al. Human gut microbiome viewed across age and geography. Nature. 2012;**486**:222-227

[67] Jost T, Lacroix C, Braegger C, Chassard C. Impact of human milk bacteria and oligosaccharides on neonatal gut microbiota establishment and gut health. Nutrition Reviews. 2015;**73**:426-437

[68] Butel M-J, Waligora Dupriet A-J, Wydau-Dematteis S. The developing gut microbiota and its consequences for health. Journal of Developmental Origins of Health and Disease. 2018;**1**:8. DOI: 10.1017/S2040174418000119

[69] Kuzniewicz MW, Wi S, Qian Y, et al. Prevalence and neonatal factors associated with autism spectrum disorders in preterm infants. The Journal of Pediatrics. 2014;**164**:20-25

[70] Kanherkar RR, Bhatia-Dey N, Csoka AB. Epigentics across the human lifespan. Frontiers in Cell and Development Biology. 2014;**2**:1-19

[71] Hochberg Z, Feil R, Constancia M, et al. Child health, developmental plasticity, and epigenetic programming. Endocrine Reviews. 2011;**32**:159-224

[72] Ghantous A, Hernandez-Vargas H, Bymes G, et al. Characterizing the epigenome as a key component of the fetal exposome in evaluating *in utero* exposures and childhood cancer risk. Mutagenesis. 2015;**30**:733-742

[73] Ladd-Acosta C, Shu C, Lee BK, et al. Presence of an epigenetic signature of prenatal cigarette smoke exposure in childhood. Environmental Research. 2017;**144**(Pt A):139-148

[74] Barouki R, Melen E, Herceg Z, et al. Epigenetics as a mechanism linking developmental exposures to long-term toxicity. Environment International. 2018;**114**:77-86.s

[75] Barua S, Kuizon S, Junaid MA. Folic acid supplementation in pregnancy and implications in health and disease. Journal of Biomedical Science. 2014;**21**:77-85

[76] Crider KS, Yang TP, Berry RJ, et al. Folate and DNA methylation: A review of molecular mechanisms and the evidence for folate's role. Advances in Nutrition. 2012;**3**:21-38

[77] Joubert BR, den Dekker HT, Felix JF, et al. Maternal plasma folate impact differential DNA methylation in an epigenome-wide meta-analysis of newborns. Nature Communications. 2016;7:10577

[78] Amarasekera M, Martino D, Ashley S, et al. Genome-wide DNA methylation profiling identifies a folate-sensitive region of differential methylation upstream of *ZFP57*-impreinting regulator in humans. The FASEB Journal. 2014;**28**:4068-4076

[79] Steegers-Theunissen RP, Obermann-Borst SA, Kremer D, et al. Periconceptional maternal folic acid use of 400 μg per day is related to increased methylation of the *IGF2* gene in the very young child. PLoS One. 2009;**4**:e7845

[80] Ba Y, Yu H, Liu F, et al. Relationship of folate, vitamin B12 and methylation

of insulin-like growth factor-II in maternal and cord blood. European Journal of Clinical Nutrition. 2011;**65**:480-485

[81] Anderson CM, Gillespe SL, Thiele DK, et al. Effects of maternal vitamin D supplementation on maternal and infant epigenome. Breastfeeding Medicine. 2018;**13**:371-380

[82] Eid A, Zawai N. Consequences of lead exposure, and its emerging role as an epigenetic modifier in the aging brain. Neurotoxicology. 2016;**56**:254-261

[83] Bommarito P, Martin E, Fry RC. Effects of prenatal exposure to endocrine disruptors and toxic metals on the fetal epigenome. Epigenomics. 2017;**9**:333-350

[84] Heijmans BT, Tobi EW, Stein AD, et al. Persistent epigenetic differences associated with prenatal exposure to famine in humans. PNAS. 2008;**105**:17046-17049

[85] DeVries A, Donata V. The neonatal methylome as a gatekeeper in the trajectory to childhood asthma. Epigenetics. 2017;**9**:585-593

Section 2

Factors Influencing Maternal Decision on Infant Feeding Methods

Chapter 2

Breastfeeding in Normal Newborn: Basic Concepts

Jayashree Purkayastha

Abstract

Breastfeeding is a complete nutrition for the baby and beneficial to the baby and the mother. Mothers should be prepared for breastfeeding and motivated antenatally. Breastfeeding should be initiated within 1 h of normal delivery and 4 h of Caesarean section. In the first 2 days, colostrum is secreted which is highly immunogenic to the baby. Mature milk comes by day 10 of life. Foremilk is rich in protein and vitamins, while hindmilk is rich in fat. Proper technique should be followed for successful breastfeeding. Reflexes in the mother while breastfeeding are prolactin and oxytocin reflexes, while reflexes in the baby are rooting, sucking and swallowing. In case of early discharge from the hospital, adequacy of breastfeeding should be checked at 3–5 days of life. Breastfeeding develops bonding between the baby and the mother and promotes brain growth of the baby. Human milk is suitable for the baby and contains less protein and minerals than cow's milk and has less solute load for immature kidneys of the baby. Breastfeeding should be on demand, minimum eight times per day. The common feeding problems in the mother are flat or inverted nipple, sore nipple, engorgement of breasts, and mastitis which should be prevented.

Keywords: breastfeeding, breastmilk, benefits, term baby, mother

1. Introduction

Breastfeeding is a birthright of every baby, and also it is the right of every mother to breastfeed her baby. Breastfeeding is a complete nutrition for the baby and has several advantages to the baby and the mother. Breastfeeding (colostrum) has so much benefit for the baby especially immunologically that it is called the first vaccine for the baby. Breastfeeding is hypoallergenic and safe to the baby. It is sterile, hygienic and also economical. Breastfeeding is the saviour of the infant from respiratory and diarrhoeal morbidity and mortality especially in the developing and underdeveloped countries. It relieves a lot of economic burden for the poor countries [1]. In low-income and middle-income countries, only 37% of the babies less than 6 months are exclusively breastfed [2]. Breastfeeding helps in brain growth and improves the intelligence quotient (IQ) of the children and thus benefits the country as a whole [3]. Breastfeeding reduces mortality and morbidity of children under 5 years of age especially in developing and underdeveloped countries. Breastfeeding enhances the bond between the mother and the child, provides tender loving care to the child and keeps the mother happy.

IntechOpen

2. Physiology of lactation

Stage 1: The mammary gland is developed to produce milk as colostrum 12 weeks prior to parturition, but colostrum secretion is inhibited by the raised progesterone levels.

Stage 2: Milk production occurs after delivery due to the decrease in progesterone and the increase in prolactin levels. By the second or third day, milk production depends on suckling of the baby.

Stage 3: Mature milk production starts after 10 days of delivery and is the third stage of lactogenesis. The lactogenic effect of prolactin is modulated by the complex interplay of pituitary, thyroid, ovarian, adrenal and pancreatic hormones [4].

2.1 Preparing mothers for breastfeeding

During the last trimester of antenatal care, the mother's nipples should be checked. In case of flat nipple or retracted nipple, oil massage and manipulation to make the nipples conducive to breastfeeding should be done. The mother should be given healthy diet, green leafy vegetables, fruits, eggs, fish (omega 3 fatty acid) and plenty of fluids. She should take extra 300 cal and 15 g of protein during the antenatal period and extra 500 cal and 25 g of protein during the lactation period [5].

2.2 Initiation of breastfeeding

Breastfeeding should be initiated as early as possible after delivery preferably within 1 h after normal delivery and 4 h after Caesarean section [5]. The baby is biologically active immediately after delivery after which the baby goes into sleep and there is difficulty in establishment of breastfeeding; hence breastfeeding should be initiated early. Immediately after delivery, he/she should be put on the mother's abdomen, crawl to the breast and suckle at the breast; this method helps in early initiation of breastfeeding. Early skin-to-skin contact, putting the baby in mother's abdomen helps in early initiation of breastfeeding [6]. Keeping the baby with the mother in the same room is called 'rooming in', keeping him/her in the same bed with his/her mother is called 'bedding in' and keeping him/her in his/her mother's abdomen is called 'mothering in' [5].

2.3 Types of breastmilk

In the first 2 days, colostrum is secreted which is rich in lymphocytes, IgA and antibodies; the colostrum secreted is 10–40 ml/day which is sufficient for a term baby and does not require any supplementation. No prelacteal feeds should be given because these can cause infection and delay in establishment of breastfeeding. The baby should be well supported while breastfeeding, and the mother may require help in the first few days. Both the mother and the baby should be comfortable while breastfeeding. A healthy baby will empty the breast within 20 min, and alternating the breasts used for each feed is advised. The baby should completely empty the breast on the one side in order to get adequate hindmilk. Foremilk is the initial milk which is rich in vitamins, proteins, sugar, mineral and fluid, while hindmilk contains fat. Hence foremilk only satisfies the thirst, and the baby needs to get adequate hindmilk to get adequate calories and to satisfy hunger. If a baby does not empty the breast each feed, he/she does not get hindmilk and hence does not get nutritional requirement and feels hungry very fast and does not gain adequate weight. Transitional milk is secreted in the first 10 days followed by mature milk. Milk production increases for the first 6 months and then plateaus off. Average milk secreted is 500–800 ml/day [5].

2.4 Technique of breastfeeding

The correct technique should be followed for successful breastfeeding. The mother should touch the angle of the baby's mouth with the nipple; rooting reflex causes the baby to open the mouth and take in the nipple and the areola into the mouth.

Good attachment: Signs of good attachment are as follows: the baby's chin should be touching the breast, the mouth should be wide open, the lower lip should be turned outwards, the upper areola should be visible and the lower areola covered (**Figure 1**). He/she should suckle at the areola and not at the nipple so that the tongue is under the lactiferous sinuses and the nipple against the palate. He/she should form an adequate seal around the nipple and areola to eject the milk from lactiferous sinuses [5].

Good positioning: The baby should be turned towards the mother; his/her head, body and buttocks should be well supported and in straight line; his/her abdomen should be against his/her mother's abdomen [7].

Burping: When the baby sucks the breast, air goes in which causes colic, regurgitation and abdominal distension; hence burping is necessary. Burping is done by putting the baby on the left shoulder and gently patting his/her back or by making him/her sit on his/her mother's lap with support and gently patting the back [7].

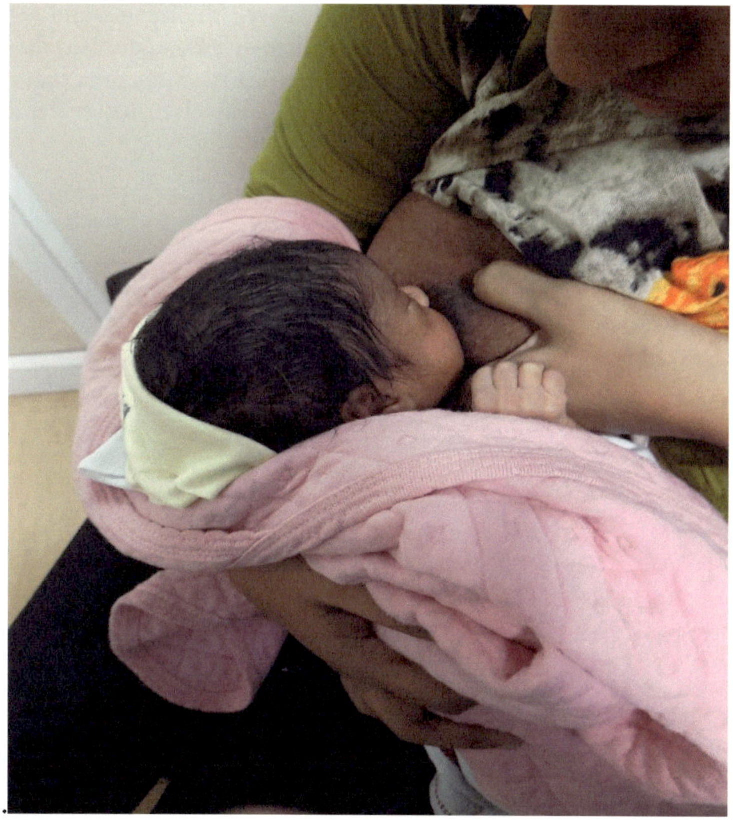

Figure 1.
Correct technique of breastfeeding (cradle hold).

2.5 Various positions of breastfeeding

Cradle hold: Mother positions the infant's head at or near the antecubital space at the level of her nipple with her arm supporting the infant's body and her other hand is free to hold the breast (**Figure 2**).

Cross cradle hold: Useful in preterm and babies with fractured clavicle. Mother holds the head with the hand opposite the side on which the infant will feed and supports the infant's body across her lap with her arm. The other hand is free to hold the breast.

Football hold: This method avoids pressure on Caesarean incision and helps in heavy breasts. Mother supports the infant's head and neck with her hand with the infant's body resting on pillows alongside her hip.

Side lying position: This position avoids pressure on episiotomy or abdominal incision and helps the mother to rest while feeding. She lies on her side and her upper hand is used to position her breast. Pillows can be put behind her back and between her legs to provide comfort. A small blanket or towel can be placed over the abdominal incision to protect from the infants' movement (**Table 1**) [8].

2.5.1 Reflexes in the mother while breastfeeding

Prolactin reflex: This is the milk production reflex; when the baby suckles at the breast, it causes sensory nerves to be stimulated which stimulates the anterior pituitary to secrete prolactin which helps in the production of milk for the next feed.

Oxytocin reflex: When the baby suckles at the breast, stimulation of posterior pituitary secretes oxytocin which contracts the myoepithelial cells and helps in the ejection of milk; this reflex is also called **let down reflex** because when the mother feeds the baby from one breast and this reflex is acting, then there will be breastmilk secretion from the other breast also, which is called drip milk. This

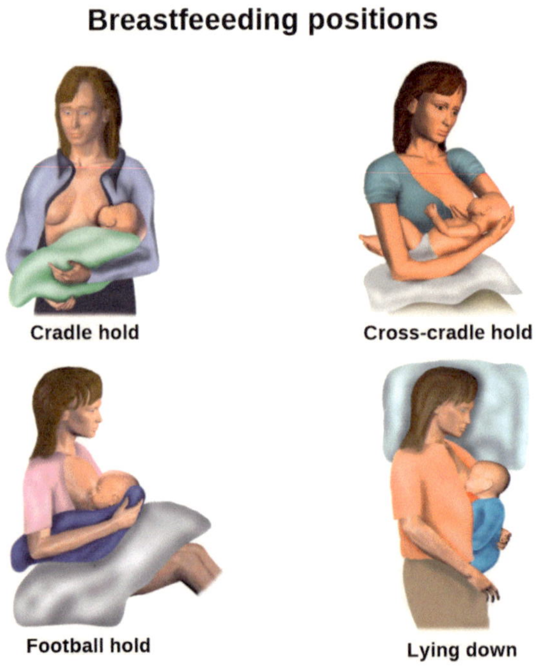

Figure 2.
Various positions of breastfeeding (taken from toko.semuada.com).

Positions	Elements positive	Elements negative
Cradle hold	Classic position	Head tends to wobble
Cross cradle hold	Provides good head control	Least familiar
Football or clutch hold	For LBW, minimum head control, avoids Caesarean incision	Teaching required
Side lying	Minimises fatigue	Chances of smothering

Table 1.
Various positions for breastfeeding.

reflex if present tells us that mother's milk is adequate. Oxytocin reflex is usually affected by the mother's mental status; if she is relaxed, calm and happy, oxytocin reflex is augmented on the other hand; if she is depressed and sad, oxytocin reflex is inhibited; for successful breastfeeding, the mother should be relaxed, calm and happy [5].

2.5.2 Reflexes in the baby

Rooting reflex: When the mother's nipple touches the angle of the mouth and then the baby opens the mouth and tries to latch at the breast, this is called rooting reflex.

Sucking reflex: The baby suckles at the areola when the nipple and the areola are put inside the mouth.

Swallowing reflex: The baby sucks and then swallows. The synchrony of respiration with sucking and swallowing takes place at 34 weeks of gestation. Babies born at or after 34 weeks of gestation can only successfully breastfeed. The rhythm is usually suck, suck, suck, pause and then swallow [5].

2.6 Adequacy of breastmilk

How to know if breastmilk is sufficient or not? In the first week of life, there will be weight loss; in an exclusively breastfed term baby, about 5–7% of birthweight is lost in the first week especially by 48–72 h of birth [9]. A term baby usually regains birthweight, on average, by 8.3 days of life [9] and starts gaining minimum ½ ounce/day for the first 3 months [10]. Hence after the first week of life, we know that breastmilk is adequate by observing adequate weight gain, five to six times, pale-coloured urine per day and golden yellow colour stools, and then baby should sleep after each feed. Also when the mother is breastfeeding from one breast, if milk drips from the other breast, it is suggestive of adequacy of milk, and the milk that drips from the other breast is called drip milk. Drip milk is low in energy and fat content. If the baby is not gaining adequate weight and urine output is less after the third day of life, it is suggestive of inadequate breastmilk; the baby needs to attend a paediatrician to prevent complications like hypernatraemic dehydration [10]. However it should be remembered that in the first 2 days of life, only colostrum is secreted which is less in amount; hence urine output may be very less so much so that we can wait for 48 h for the first passage of urine. There is no need to give any complementary feeds to the baby in the first 2–3 days when colostrum is less because whatever colostrum is there, it is enough to meet the nutritional needs of a term baby, and a term baby also contains enough stores of glycogen. In case of early discharge from the hospital exclusively, breastfed babies should be seen by a paediatrician on the third to fifth day of life to check the adequacy of breastmilk and establishment of lactation [10].

2.7 Benefits of breastmilk

2.7.1 Benefits to the baby

1. It is a complete nutrition for the baby till 6 months of age. It is easily digestible due to the presence of lipase and whey proteins.

2. Breastmilk contains anti-infective properties, antibodies, IgA and lactobacilli which protect the baby from diarrhoea, respiratory tract infection, otitis media and necrotizing enterocolitis.

3. Breastmilk is hypoallergenic and reduces disorders like asthma and eczema in breastfed babies.

4. **Biochemical benefits:** Protein is predominantly whey protein which contains alpha lactalbumin and lactoferrin. Lactalbumin is rich in tryptophan which is a precursor of serotonin and plays an important role as neurotransmitter. Lactoferrin helps in the absorption of iron and zinc and is bacteriostatic. Calcium phosphorus ratio is more than 2 and helps in calcium absorption. Protein content is less which provides less solute load to the baby's kidneys.

5. **Microbiological benefits:** It is sterile and there is less chance of contamination. Lactoferrin is bacteriostatic and inhibits E. coli growth in gut; lactoferrin binds with iron and makes it unavailable to E. coli. Peroxidases and lipases kill bacteria. The bifidus factor promotes the growth of lactobacilli. Bile salt-stimulated lipase (BSSL) kills amoeba and Giardia. Deficiency of para-aminobenzoic acid (PABA) in breastmilk prevents the growth of malarial parasite.

6. **Immunological benefits:** Breastmilk supplies passive immunity to the baby. It contains macrophages, lysozymes and complements, T lymphocytes and B lymphocytes. Secretory IgA provides surface immunity to GI tract and respiratory tract.

7. **Psychological benefits:** Breastfeeding promotes bonding between the mother and the baby. Breastfeeding provides maternal warmth, closeness and comfort to the baby.

8. **Better IQ:** Breastfed babies have higher intelligence quotient than formula-fed babies and have enhanced visual development. Breastmilk contains long-chain fatty acids like arachidonic acid (AHA) and docosahexaenoic acid (DHA), lactose and sialic acid which promote brain growth. Breastmilk contains choline, taurine and iodine which promote brain growth.

9. Breastfed babies have less risk of developing diabetes mellitus, high blood pressure, obesity, heart attack and certain cancers in adult life [5, 11–13].

2.7.2 Benefits to the mother

1. Breastfeeding releases oxytocin which helps in involution of the uterus which leads to less chance of postpartum haemorrhage.

2. Mothers who breastfeed have lactational amenorrhoea and have less chance of conception during that period. Night feeds especially help in preventing conception during lactational amenorrhea.

3. Breastfeeding is convenient, economical and readily available at the desired temperature.

4. Mothers develop a close bond with the baby; they feel relaxed and happy to take care of their baby.

5. Mothers regain their prepregnancy weight earlier than in those mothers who formula feed their babies because the energy stored during pregnancy is lost during lactation.

6. Mothers who breastfeed their babies have less chance of developing breast cancer and ovarian cancer [5, 11–13].

2.8 Breastmilk and brain growth

Breastmilk contains arachidonic acid (AHA), docosahexaenoic acid (DHA), high contents of amino acids like cysteine and taurine, choline, iodine, zinc, lactose and oligosaccharides which promotes maturation, myelination and synaptogenesis of the human brain [3].

2.9 Composition of breastmilk and cow's milk

Breastmilk contains less protein and solute load which are suitable for the baby and their immature kidneys. Cow's milk protein is predominantly casein, whereas breastmilk contains whey protein which is easily digestible. It is mainly lactalbumin and lactoferrin. Casein to whey protein ratio is 40:60 in human milk and 80:20 in cow's milk. Cow's milk contains lactoglobulin which is the cause of intolerance to cow's milk. Lactobacilli and lactic acid are probiotics which help in digestion in human milk. Nonprotein nitrogen in human milk like urea, amino acids, choline, creatinine, uric acid, ammonia and N-acetylglutamine are bioactive factors which are not present in cow's milk. Breastmilk is rich in long-chain polyunsaturated fatty acid (PUFA) like eicosapentaenoic acid (EPA) and docosahexaenoic acid (DHA). Cow's milk is rich in saturated fats. The polyunsaturated/saturated fat ratio is 1.2:1 in breastmilk compared to 1:2 in cow's milk. Carbohydrate in breastmilk is lactose which is double in content in breastmilk than in cow's milk and is suitable for brain growth and for the development of normal GI flora in babies. Vitamins like K and D are deficient in breastmilk. Especially in vitamin D-deficient mothers, breastmilk contains less vitamin D, and hence vitamin D supplementation in normal newborn exclusively breastfed babies is essential. Vitamin K is given to all babies after birth to prevent haemorrhagic disease of newborn. Minerals are less in breastmilk, but bioavailability is better in breastmilk than in cow's milk. Cow's milk contains high levels of electrolytes and hence high solute load and is not suitable for immature kidneys of babies [5, 12] (**Table 2**).

2.10 Breastfeeding schedule

In a normal term baby, breastfeeding should be done as and when baby demands. Usually after every 2–3 h, the baby will wake up and cry for feeds; this is called demand feeding. Some babies might sleep for a long duration usually in the first few

Nutrition	Human milk	Cow's milk
Calories	65	67
Protein	1.1 g	3.5 g
Lactose	7.4 g	4.5 g
Fat	3.5 g	3.5 g
Calcium	35 mg	140 mg
Phosphorus	15 mg	90 mg
Magnesium	4 mg	12 mg
Electrolytes (meq/L)		
Sodium	6.5	25
Chloride	12	29
Potassium	14	35
Osmolality (mosm/L)	290	350
Vitamins		
Vitamin A (μg)	53	34
Vitamin D (IU)	0.4–10	0.3–4
Vitamin E (mg)	0.2	
Vitamin K1 (μg)	0.3	0.7
Vitamin C (mg)	4.3	1.8
Thiamine (B1) (μg)	16	42
Riboflavin (B2) (μg)	43	157
Niacin (μg)	172	85
Vitamin B6 (μg)	11	58
Folic acid (μg)	0.18	0.23
Vitamin B12 (μg)	0.18	0.4
Biotin (μg)	2	22
Choline (mg)	1.3	1.2
Taurine (mg)	5	0.5
Carnitine (mg)	0.8	1
Iron (mg)	0.05–0.2	0.1–0.3
Iodine (mg)	7	21
Copper (mg)	0.04	0.03
Zinc (mg)	0.53	0.38

Table 2.
Human milk versus cow's milk composition per 100 ml [5, 12].

days after birth; these babies should be awakened and fed if the gap exceeds more than 3 h. Some babies sleep off after few minutes of suckling; they should be aroused by tickling at the ears and flicking the sole, or the mother should try to withdraw the nipple and then the baby starts suckling again [12]. Usually a normal term baby requires 15–20 min to empty one breast; he/she should be allowed to completely empty one breast so that he/she gets both foremilk and the hindmilk, which is required for the satiety of hunger and weight gain. If the baby sleeps off after a few mins, he/she should be aroused and then start suckling again and complete the feed [12]. Breastfeeding should be continued till 2 years of age because the maximum growth and myelination of the brain take place in the first 2 years of life [5]. After 6 months of age, weaning should be started which is done by introducing semisolids or complementary feeds to the diet along with breastfeeding. After 6 months of life, the baby becomes interested in his/her surroundings and shows interest when adults take food; breastmilk output of the mother is not sufficient to meet the needs of the baby, and hence semisolid diet according to the regional availability may be introduced. If weaning is not started by 6 months of age, it might lead to malnutrition. An exclusively breastfed term baby does not require multivitamin supplementation; however the baby may be given vitamin D supplementation for a period of 6 months [10].

2.11 Immunobiology of breastmilk

Colostrum is very rich in secretory IgA (sIgA) which protects the mucosal lining of GI tract and respiratory tract and contains lymphocytes and macrophages. After 2–3 days, colostrum is replaced by transitional breastmilk which contains less amount of sIgA than colostrum. SIgA are produced in the mammary gland by the plasma cells that are derived from gut-associated lymphoid tissue (GALT) and bronchus-associated lymphoid tissue (BALT) [5]. Breastmilk contains sIgA and also IgM antibodies. IgM antibodies are transmitted from the mother to the baby by breastmilk; IgM antibodies usually do not cross the placenta and are not transferred from the mother to the baby via the placenta [12]. Breastmilk also contains IgG antibodies, lymphocytes, polymorph, macrophages and plasma cells and nonspecific humoral factors like lysozyme, oligosaccharides, lactoferrin and lactoperoxidase. Probiotics in breastmilk protects the gut from enteric pathogens. It also contains antiviral and anti-staphylococcal factors [12].

2.12 Common feeding problems in the mother

2.12.1 Flat or inverted nipple

If the nipple is flat, the areola and the nipple should be brought out to form the teat; otherwise the baby cannot latch a flat nipple. Occasionally while trying to pull out the nipple, it goes deeper into the breast and this is called inverted nipple; in this case the baby finds difficulty in latching. Nipple protractility test (nipple should be capable of being pulled out) should be done in the last trimester of pregnancy [14]. The nipple might get corrected as the baby sucks. In case of problem, syringe technique should be tried (**Figure 3**). Supple cups or silicone nipple can be used over flat or inverted nipple to form a teat so that the baby can suckle.

2.12.2 Prevention of engorgement of breasts

Usually by days 2–3, milk production increases, and if the baby is not put for suckling, the breasts get engorged. If the breasts get engorged, then the nipple and areola becomes hard and baby does not suck at the breast. To relieve breast engorgement, breasts have to be emptied; this can be done by putting the baby for frequent suckling at the breast or by emptying the breast using breast pump. Warm packs applied to breasts or a warm shower before feeding combined with massage helps to relieve the congestion [8].

2.12.3 Prevention of sore nipples

This may occur from strong sucking action of the baby if his/her position is not correct, i.e. if he/she sucks at the nipple instead of the areola; correct breastfeeding

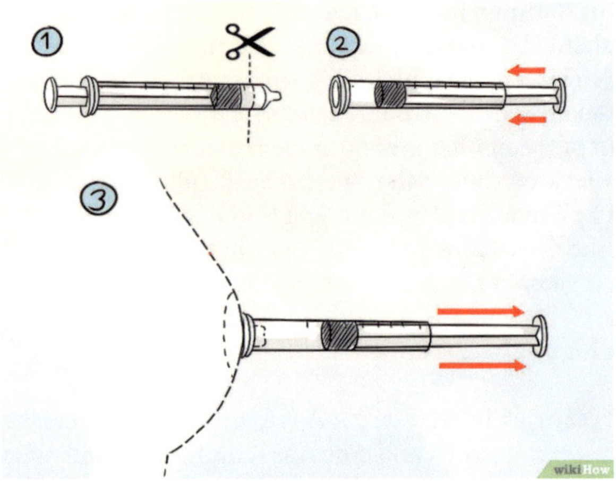

Figure 3.
Syringe technique for flat and inverted nipple (taken from Wikihow.com).

technique can prevent sore nipples. The baby should not be forcefully removed from sucking at the breast, but instead a finger can be introduced to break the suction and then remove him/her; he/she should not be allowed to suck for a long time after the breast is emptied; the nipple should not be allowed to remain wet from leaking milk. The mother can keep the nipple exposed to air for 10–15 min after breastfeeding or apply vitamin E lotion, coconut oil and lanolin to prevent soreness. While cleaning the nipples, she should avoid using soap and use only warm water. In case of sore nipple or cracked nipple, nipple shells or nipple shields can be used to allow the baby to suckle and to prevent the mother from pain [7].

2.12.4 Blocked ducts

Sometimes a segment of the breast becomes hard due to blocked ducts; in this case proper massage and warm packs with emptying of the breast helps, and if blocked ducts are not treated, it leads to mastitis [5]. Sometimes due to incorrect technique and engorgement of breasts if not treated, the mother may develop mastitis (non-infective); in this condition mothers should be given analgesia (paracetamol) prior to feeds, and the baby should be put for suckling; if baby cannot be put for suckling at the breast due to pain, breasts must be emptied by using breast pump; the mother should take bed rest and plenty of fluids orally. In case the mother develops breast abscess, antibiotics should be given for 10–14 days. Breastfeeding can be continued from the affected breast if there is no pus discharge from the nipple [15]. Breast abscess might require drainage. Candidal infection: sometimes mothers may experience excruciating pain while feeding the baby; if the baby has oral thrush, 1% gentian violet clotrimazole mouth paint may be applied over the nipple and inside the baby's mouth. Mothers may require systemic antifungal like fluconazole in severe cases [16]. Psychological counselling for the mother is necessary in these cases of feeding problems. A mother needs constant support and guidance in these cases [5].

2.13 Breastfeeding when the mother is ill

A mother can breastfeed her baby in case of fever, rhinitis, respiratory tract infection, diarrheal diseases and asthma provided she is not very sick and unable to breastfeed. In case of respiratory tract infections, she should wear mask while breastfeeding. If the mother is unable to breastfeed, expressed breastmilk (EBM) can be given through cup and spoon. Breastmilk can be expressed using manual or electric breast pump. Bottle feeds should not be used because it creates nipple confusion in the baby and the baby will refuse to take breastfeeding. Bottle feeding is easier and needs less energy, and henceforth the baby becomes lazy and refuses breastfeeding [12]. If the mother has mastitis, she can breastfeed from the unaffected breast and also from the affected breast if there is no pus discharge from the nipple of affected site [15]. In case of UTI and tuberculosis (if sputum is negative), breastfeeding can be given. In case of hepatitis B-positive mother, the baby should be given hepatitis B immunoglobulin and hepatitis B vaccine after birth, and breastfeeding can be continued [5]. In case of HIV-positive mother, the **WHO** recommends to continue breastfeeding in developing countries because in developing countries morbidity and mortality is high if the baby is not breastfed due to other infections like respiratory and diarrhoeal diseases. However in the case of higher socioeconomic status, breastfeeding can be stopped and formula feeds may be given in HIV-positive mothers. **CDC** recommends to stop breastfeeding in HIV-positive mothers [17]. In postpartum psychosis, breastfeeding may be allowed under supervision.

2.14 Contraindications to breastfeeding

Galactosemia, congenital lactose intolerance, chemotherapy, antithyroid drugs except propylthiouracil and antipsychotic drugs like lithium are contraindications for breastfeeding [5].

2.15 Breastfeeding-associated problems

2.15.1 Regurgitation of feeds

Some babies regurgitate some curdy milk precipitates (fermented milk from the stomach) after each feed; the mother should be advised to burp the baby properly to eructate the swallowed air and to make the baby lie in right lateral position with slight elevation of the head.

2.15.2 Gastrocolic reflex

Some breastfed babies may pass stool after each feed; this is not diarrhoea, and if urine output is good, then there is no dehydration and no treatment required; it is a phenomenon due to gastrocolic reflex. If the urine output is good then it is normal.

2.15.3 Evening colic

Some breastfed babies cry during the evening hours due to aerophagia. These babies can be put prone, and burping can be done which will help the air to come out and relieve the colic [12].

2.16 Breastfeeding in working mothers

Usually working mothers get 6 months of maternity leave. In the first 6 months, exclusive breastfeeding can be given and then complementary feeds should be started along with breastfeeding.

Ideally there should be a crèche near the working place for the mother to go and feed in between. There should be a private place in the working area for the mother to express her milk and give to her baby in the crèche. Expressed breastmilk can be given to the baby if the mother is away by cup and spoon [5].

2.17 Breastmilk storage

Expressed breastmilk (EBM) should be stored in a stainless steel, food grade hard plastic or glass container having a tight fitting lid. EBM can be stored at room temperature for 6 h and in the refrigerator for 24 h and in the freezer compartment of the refrigerator for 2 weeks. EBM should be thawed before feeding by running tap or lukewarm water over the container; never use boiling or hot water to thaw the milk. EBM should never be heated or microwaved because the antibodies get destroyed [18].

2.18 Medications to the lactating mothers

All drugs taken by the mother will be excreted in the milk, but the concentration of drugs in the breastmilk is less, usually less than 1%. Propylthiouracil and warfarin are safe and can be taken during breastfeeding. Antibiotics taken by the mother may cause increased stooling of the baby. Laxatives taken by the mother can cause diarrhoea in the baby; however milk of magnesia, liquid paraffin and glycerine suppositories are safe. Oral contraceptives, pyridoxine, nicotine and bromocriptine suppress lactation [5].

2.19 Delayed lactation

Some mothers with obesity, diabetes mellitus, stress, polycystic ovarian disease, postpartum haemorrhage and retained placenta may have delayed lactation. In these cases galactogogues can be given like domperidone and metoclopramide tablets. However it should be kept in mind that these drugs can cause extra pyramidal symptoms (EPS) in the mother. Domperidone has less chance of EPS and is well tolerated and can be given for 7–10 days at length [5].

2.20 Baby-friendly hospital initiative (BFHI)

The Baby-friendly Hospital Initiative (BFHI) was started in the year 1992 organised by the UNICEF and WHO. The World Alliance for Breastfeeding Action (WABA) is the global agency for the promotion of breastfeeding. The 10 steps of BFHI are as follows [5]:

1. Every hospital should have a written breastfeeding policy that is routinely communicated to all healthcare staff.

2. Train all healthcare staff in skills necessary to implement this policy.

3. Inform all pregnant women about the benefits and management of breastfeeding.

4. Help mothers to initiate breastfeeding within an hour of birth.

5. Show mothers how to breastfeed and how to maintain lactation even if they are separated from their infants.

6. Give newborn infants no food or drink other than breastmilk, unless medically indicated.

DOI: http://dx.doi.org/10.5772/intechopen.92250

7. Practise rooming-in and allow mothers and infants to remain together 24 h a day.

8. Encourage breastfeeding on demand.

9. Give no artificial teats or pacifiers (also called dummies or soothers) to breastfeeding infants.

10. Foster the establishment of breastfeeding support groups, and refer mothers to them on discharge from the hospital or clinic.

2.21 Breastfeeding week celebration

Every year breastfeeding week is celebrated from August 1 to August 7. It commemorates the Innocenti Declaration in August 1990 when the WHO, UNICEF and several other organisations came together to protect, promote and support breastfeeding. Every year there is a theme based on which it is celebrated. Breastfeeding week celebrations are organised by the WABA, UNICEF, WHO and several government and non-government organisations [19].

3. Conclusion

All mothers should be antenatally motivated for breastfeeding. Breastfeeding should be initiated within 1 h of birth. Early skin-to-skin contact helps in early initiation of breastfeeding. Correct technique of breastfeeding should be taught to the mother. Exclusive breastfeeding should be given for 6 months of age and then complementary feeds should be introduced. In low- and middle-income countries, breastfeeding not only benefits the mother and the baby but also reduces economic burden of the country. Hence we should protect, promote and support breastfeeding not only in low- and middle-income countries but also in developed countries.

Acknowledgements

I would like to acknowledge Dr. Sneha Andrade and Veronica sister for helping me take the picture of the mother while breastfeeding. I would also like to acknowledge the mother for allowing me to take the picture.

Conflict of interest

The author declares no conflict of interest.

Author details

Jayashree Purkayastha
Kasturba Medical College, MAHE, Manipal, Karnataka, India

*Address all correspondence to: jayashreepurkayastha@yahoo.com

References

[1] Rollins NC, Bhandari N, Hajeebhoy N, Horton S, Lutter CK, Martines JC, et al. Why invest, and what it will take to improve breastfeeding practices? Lancet. 2016;**387**:491-504. DOI: 10.1016/s0140-6736(15)01044-2

[2] Victoria CG, Bahl R, Barros AJ, Franca GV, Horton S, Krasevec J, et al. Breastfeeding in the 21st century: Epidemiology, mechanisms, and lifelong effect. Lancet. 2016;**387**(10017):475-490. DOI: 10.1016/s0140-6736(15)01024-7

[3] Horta BL, Loret de Mola C, Victoria CG. Breastfeeding and intelligence: A systematic review and meta-analysis. Acta Paediatrica. 2015;**104**(467):14-19. DOI: 10.1111/apa-13139

[4] Lawrence RA, Lawrence RM. Physiology of lactation. In: Breastfeeding: A Guide for the Medical Profession. 6th ed. Philadelphia: Elsevier Mosby; 2005. pp. 68-100

[5] Elizabeth KE. Infant and young child feeding (IYCF). In: Nutrition and Child Development. 4th ed. New Delhi: Paras Medical Publisher; 2010. pp. 1-22

[6] Moore ER, Bergman N, Anderson GC, Medley N. Early skin-to-skin contact for mothers and their healthy newborn infants. Cochrane Database of Systematic Reviews. 2016;(11):CD003519. DOI: 10.10002/14651858.CD003519pub4

[7] Novan JC, Broom BL. Ingalls and Salerno's Maternal and Child Health Nursing. 9th ed. Missouri: Mosby; 1999

[8] Murray SS, McKinney ES. Foundations of Maternal-Newborn and Women's Health Nursing. 5th ed. Saunders Elsevier: Missouri; 2010

[9] MacDonald DP, Ross RS, Grant L, Young D. Neonatal weight loss in breast and formula fed infants. Archives of Disease in Childhood. Fetal and Neonatal Edition. 2003;**88**(6):F472-F476

[10] Hurst N, Poupolo KM. Breastfeeding and maternal medications. In: Eichenwald EC, Hansen AR, Martin CR, Stark AR, editors. Cloherty and Stark's Manual of Neonatal Care. 8th ed. Philadelphia: Wolters Kluwer; 2017. pp. 285-288

[11] Grummer-Strawn LM, Rollins N. Summarising the health effects of breastfeeding. Acta Paediatrica. 2015;**104**(467):1-2. DOI: 10.1111/apa-13136

[12] Singh M. Feeding and nutrition. In: Care of the Newborn. 7th ed. New Delhi: Sagar Publications; 2010. pp. 168-182

[13] Guideline: Protecting, Promoting and Supporting Breastfeeding in Facilities Providing Maternity and Newborn Services. Geneva: WHO; 2017 Licence: CCBY-NC-SA3.0IGO. Available from: http://www.ncbi.nlm.nih.gov/books/NBK487819

[14] Alexander J, Campbell M. Prevalence of inverted and non protractile nipples in antenatal women who intend to breastfeed. The Breast. 1997;**6**(2):72-78

[15] Banapurmath RC, Banapurmath CS, Mallikarjuna RH, Kalliath A, Rao KT, Verghese J, et al. Successful management of breast abscess with ongoing breastfeeding. Indian Pediatrics. 1995;**32**:488-490

[16] Lawrence RA, Lawrence RM. Medical complications of the mother. In: Breastfeeding: A Guide for the Medical Profession. 6th ed. Philadelphia: Elsevier Mosby; 2005. pp. 562-568

[17] World Health Organization, United Nations Children's Fund. Updates

on HIV and Infant Feeding: The Duration of Breastfeeding and Support from Health Services to Improve Feeding Practices among Mothers Living with HIV. Geneva. World Health Organization; 2016. Available from: http://apps.who.int/iris/bitstream/10665/246260/1/9789241549707-eng.pdf?ua=1 [Accessed: 20 September 2017]

[18] Lawrence RA, Lawrence RM. The storage of human milk. Academy of breastfeeding medicine-human milk storage information for home use for healthy full term infants. In: Breastfeeding: A Guide for the Medical Profession. 6th ed. Philadelphia: Elsevier Mosby; 2005. pp. 1018-1020

[19] World Breastfeeding Week. 2019. Available from: www.waba.org.my

Chapter 3

Factors Influencing Maternal Decision-Making on Infant Feeding Practices

Whitney N. Hamilton

Abstract

The decision to formula feed or breastfeed a child typically begins with an established prenatal intention. This chapter will examine the multiple dimensions influencing maternal decision-making in regards to the feeding practices of infants including 1) individual maternal characteristics, 2) organizational factors, 3) hospital/provider recommendations, and 4) systematic/policy factors. The chapter will also examine the impact of infant feeding practices on early infant and childhood health outcomes. Research has demonstrated the benefits of breastfeeding on infants and early childhood which includes but is not limited to protection against common illnesses and infections, improved IQ, and even increased school attendance. Moreover, the World Health Assembly global nutrition objectives focus on encouraging breastfeeding support across all sectors in addition to implementing tailored community-based approaches, limiting the excessive marketing of infant formula, and enforcing supportive breastfeeding legislation. The aim of this chapter is to provide an overview of the dynamic interplay between individual, interpersonal, community, and societal factors, such as policies that impact breastfeeding rates and more specifically the health of infants.

Keywords: infant feeding, breastfeeding, health outcomes

1. Introduction

Key Points

- The World Health Organization recommends mothers exclusively breastfeed their children for the first 6 months of life and thereafter, supplement nutritious foods and breastmilk for up to 2 years and beyond in order for children and mothers to reap the optimal health benefits associated with breastfeeding.

- Despite the known health and economic benefits of breastfeeding, global breastfeeding prevalence remains an underachieved target, where less than 40% of infants are globally breastfed according to the WHO's recommendations [1].

- The World Health Assembly (WHA) has a goal of increasing the prevalence of exclusive breastfeeding to at least 50% by the year 2025 [1].

- In order to increase global breastfeeding prevalence understanding and addressing the individual maternal characteristics, community, organizational, and political factors affecting breastfeeding practices is crucial.

Breastfeeding is a child's first barrier against death and disease, providing protection against respiratory infection, gastrointestinal illness, and other adverse health outcomes [1–3]. Breastfeeding has also been associated with increased IQ, school attendance, as well as higher income in adult life [2, 3] The World Health Organization recommends infants exclusively receive breastmilk for the first 6 months of life and consume nutritionally adequate foods in addition to breastmilk for 2 years and beyond in order for children and mothers to reap the optimal health benefits associated with breastfeeding [1]. Nearly 1 million deaths of children under the age of 5 worldwide could be averted through breastfeeding alone, if families adhered to the World Health Organization's breastfeeding recommendation [2]. Improving maternal compliance to optimal breastfeeding recommendations can also reduce a mother's risk of ovarian cancer, heart disease, and diabetes and prevent approximately 20,000 maternal deaths from breast cancer alone. Breastfeeding also delays the return of the menstrual cycle which can help with birth spacing. Global adherence to optimal breastfeeding practices can lead to an array of health benefits coupled with economic benefits contributing to a worldwide economic savings of 300 billion U.S. dollars [1, 2].

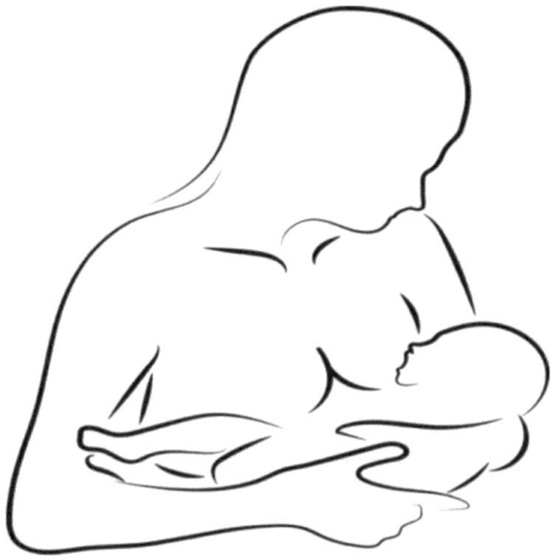

The World Health Assembly (WHA), which is the governing body of the World Health Organization, recognizes the benefits of breastfeeding and has set a goal of increasing the prevalence of exclusive breastfeeding to at least 50% by the year 2025. In addition to the WHA breastfeeding objective, the **Global Breastfeeding Collective**, a partnership of non-governmental organizations, academic institutions, and donors, led by UNICEF and WHO, seeks to work alongside WHA to accelerate progress toward reaching the breastfeeding targets and improve overall rates of breastfeeding initiation and continuation for 2 years [4]. The World Bank Investment Framework for Nutrition estimates that by reaching the WHA breastfeeding targets in 2025, would prevent over 500,000 child deaths as well as save approximately $300 billion as a result of improved child development and survival rates [5].

Despite the recognized benefits of breastfeeding, only 38% of infants worldwide are exclusively breastfed for 6 months [4]. The maternal decision on infant feeding practices begins with an established prenatal intention to breast or formula feed. Macro-level factors such as media broadcasting, infant formula marketing, and breastfeeding legislation interact with the micro-level factors which include hospitals, workplaces, and cultural norms that are supportive or discouraging to a woman's intent to breastfeed [6].

The prevalence of breastfeeding remains variable around the world due to the lack of necessary support for a mother to sustain breastfeeding [7]. Economic pressures, societal factors, and the lack of positive media coverage on breastfeeding has resulted in a cultural shift that does not fully support breastfeeding and are cited reasons for reduced breastfeeding rates globally [8]. The excessive marketing, support of, and reliance on infant formula has created a new culture and standard for infant feeding practices [8].

2. Breastfeeding prevalence

As aforementioned, the overall rate of exclusive breastfeeding for infants under 6 months of age is slightly less than 40% despite the known benefits of breastfeeding [4]. However, the least developed countries have experienced the greatest improvement in exclusive breastfeeding rates, where exclusive breastfeeding prevalence at 6 months increased from 38% in 2000 to 50% in 2012 [9]. In such developing countries a majority of infants are also still breastfeeding at 1 year in contrast to the approximate 20% in developed countries and the less than 1% still breastfeeding in the UK [3, 4]. According to the World Health Organization, only 23 countries have achieved at least 60% of infants less than 6 months being exclusively breastfed and nearly 40% of countries have breastfeeding initiation rates above 80%. In Africa, approximately 70% of countries have extended duration rates of continued breastfeeding for at least 1 year. In contrast, only four countries in the Americas have reached such high rates of breastfeeding duration at 1 year. The duration of breastfeeding for 2 years dramatically drops to 45% and no country in the Americas experiences a continued breastfeeding duration of 2 years [4].

The high initiation rate and reduced duration rate suggest many mothers intend to breastfeed but may face barriers to continue breastfeeding. The most commonly cited breastfeeding barriers as indicated in research include misinformation regarding the specific benefits of breastfeeding, social norms, lack of spousal and family support, child-birth complications, maternal employment, and lack of healthcare provider breastfeeding recommendations [10]. **The Global Breastfeeding Collective's Call to Action** highlights seven priorities to improve global breastfeeding prevalence including 1) funding breastfeeding programs, 2) eliminating the promotion of infant formula, 3) enacting legislation to protect the rights of breastfeeding women, 4) providing breastfeeding support and maternity services, 5) improving community support for breastfeeding, 6) developing systems to monitor and improve breastfeeding programs and 7) disseminating accurate information on the significance of breastfeeding (see **Table 1**) [11].

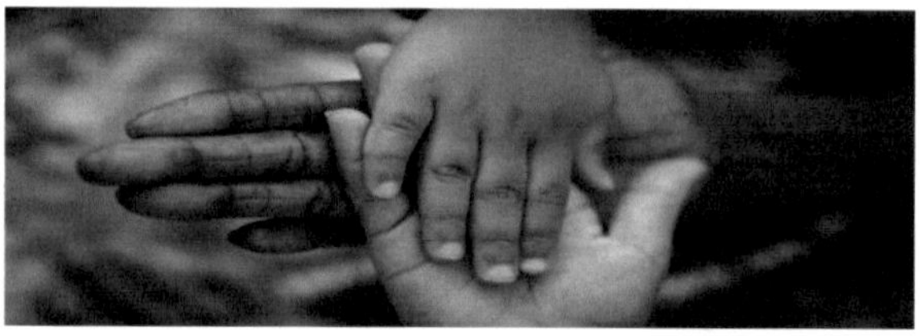

Exclusive breastfeeding	The practice of giving an infant only breastmilk for the first 6 months of life (no additional food or water) [1].
Optimal breastfeeding	Exclusively breastfeeding an infant for the first 6 months of life followed by continued breastfeeding supplementary to nutritious food for 2 years of age and beyond [1].

Table 1.
Key breastfeeding terminology.

3. Determinants of breastfeeding in developing and developed countries

Unique factors exist in developing and developed countries that influence breastfeeding behaviors. Research illustrates child and maternal morbidities such as infant colic and maternal infection are critical factors influencing breastfeeding in developing countries in contrast to developed countries. In developing countries, mothers who experience breast infections, swelling, pain, and/or chronic conditions or had infants with congenital or acquired disease were less likely to breastfeed [12, 13]. Environmental factors also have a great influence on breastfeeding in developing countries due to the limited availability of electricity to refrigerate breastmilk and the fear of contamination due to unsanitary feeding environments prevalent in some underdeveloped areas [12, 13]. Unlike developing countries that face major challenges associated directly with maternal and child health, major influences of breastfeeding practices in developed countries stem from health systems, political, and societal factors. However, in both developing and developed countries there is an interaction between individual maternal characteristics, interpersonal, community, and societal factors, such as policies and legislation that impact a mother's decision to start and continue breastfeeding [12, 13]. It may be difficult for mothers to sustain breastfeeding even after initiating due to sociodemographic, social-cultural, and systematic factors that are not supportive of breastfeeding practices (see **Figure 1** below).

3.1 Maternal characteristics

Correlates of breastfeeding initiation and duration as indicated in research include maternal marital status, vaginal delivery, previous live birth, multiple live birth (plurality), smoking and drinking habits, prenatal care within the first trimester, conversation with a healthcare provider about breastfeeding, and birth intendedness [14, 15]. Additional factors associated with breastfeeding behaviors include maternal age, race and ethnicity, level of educational

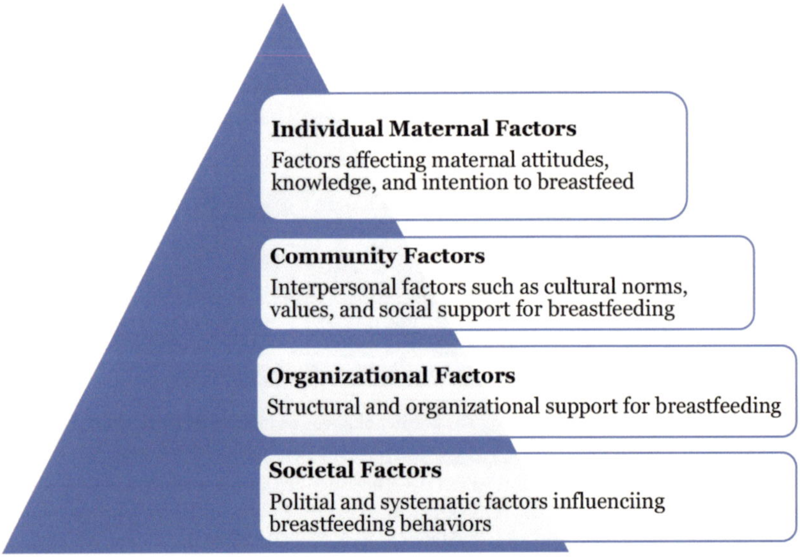

Figure 1.
Social determinants of breastfeeding.

attainment, employment status, annual household income, and Body Mass Index (BMI) [14, 15]. Teenage mothers, specifically those who had a cesarean section, experienced postpartum depression, and/or perceived an inadequate supply of breastmilk reported a shorter duration of exclusive breastfeeding. The ethnicity of mothers also has a significant association with duration of exclusive breastfeeding, which could be related to the traditions of various ethnicities in addition to religious recommendations and views [14, 15]. For example, in the U.S., black women have the lowest breastfeeding initiation and duration rates of all ethnicities [14]. The racial breastfeeding disparity among black women in the U.S. persists due to several cultural misperceptions. For instance, a common cultural belief prevalent in the black community is that the addition of cereal to an infant's bottle will help the infant sleep longer [16]. Furthermore, a mother's pre-existing health issues including obesity, experiencing multiple pregnancy complications, or giving birth to a premature child were also associated with a shorter duration of exclusive breastfeeding [15]. A mother's lack of knowledge regarding breastfeeding, limited breastfeeding guidance, poor family and social support are also associated with a lack or shorter duration of exclusive breastfeeding.

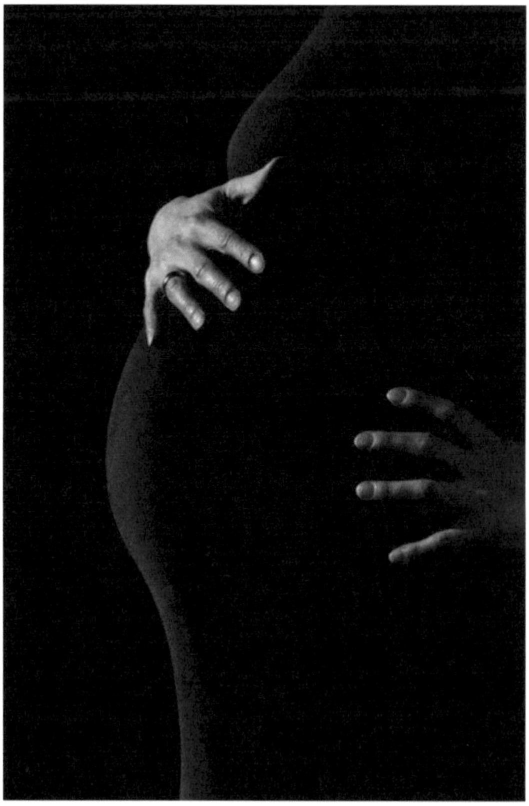

In contrast, the likelihood of breastfeeding is higher among mothers who received a high school diploma, married, and older at childbirth. Married mothers are more likely to breastfeed because they are more likely to receive spousal support that helps overcome breastfeeding challenges. Other factors that significantly improve the duration of exclusive breastfeeding include a singleton pregnancy, breastfeeding friendly birthing facility, natural vaginal delivery, babies' proper weight gain during breastfeeding, and the calmness of the infant [15].

3.2 Community factors (cultural values and norms)

3.2.1 Common misperceptions and attitudes toward breastfeeding

The following are actual quotes from various members of global communities illustrating common misconceptions associated with breastfeeding [17].

'If you tell them to exclusively breastfeed up to six months they disagree as they claim the breast will sag.' (FGD, Community Health Workers, Viwandani)

'The others will tell her that the child is big and ask why she is still breastfeeding ... So 'the duration of breastfeeding is maybe one year and most of them don't want to exceed' (KII, TBA, Korogocho).

'They mostly have fear of breastfeeding, this fear makes them not breastfeed because of fear of being seen breastfeeding since they are still young, and to remove the breast in public will be difficult.' (KII, Youth Leader, Korogocho)

Cultural attitudes, lack of public acceptance, and social norms which sexualize breasts may discourage women from breastfeeding in public [10]. Interventions promoting behavior change with regards to breastfeeding should focus on dispelling the negative cultural beliefs and practices that result in suboptimal breastfeeding practices. Infant feeding practices are strongly influenced by family members and spouses who may not be well informed about optimal breastfeeding practices. In some communities, breastfeeding in public is perceived as a culturally unacceptable practice. Therefore, disseminating tailored communication messages addressing prevailing misperceptions that build on the positive aspects of breastfeeding while involving spouses and other family members is also critical in shifting the negative perceptions of breastfeeding.

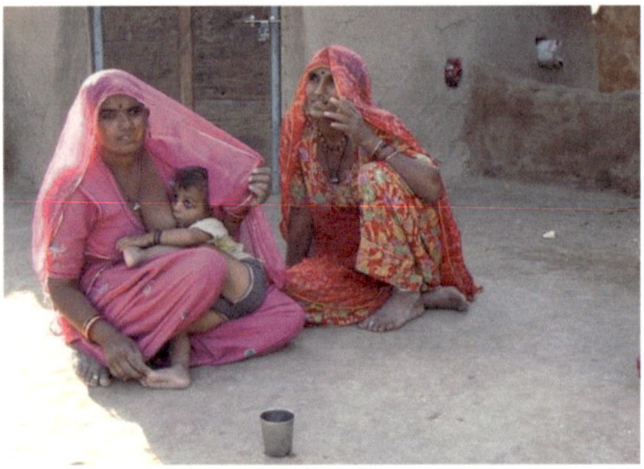

3.3 Organizational factors

3.3.1 Hospital/provider recommendations

Pediatricians, obstetricians, and other healthcare workers are usually the most trusted and credible source on infant health and nutrition [18]. The practices of maternity hospitals regarding breastfeeding and the recommendation of health providers contribute to a mother's decision to breastfeed. New mothers may lack the confidence or relevant knowledge regarding breastfeeding and health workers can play an important role by providing lactation guidance and helping to resolve challenges [1]. Lactation issues that may arise can be addressed through breastfeeding support and counseling. Thus, healthcare workers should be adequately trained to support breastfeeding and help mothers manage common lactation barriers and challenges. The support of healthcare providers enables women to attain the confidence and skills needed to successfully and optimally breastfeed.

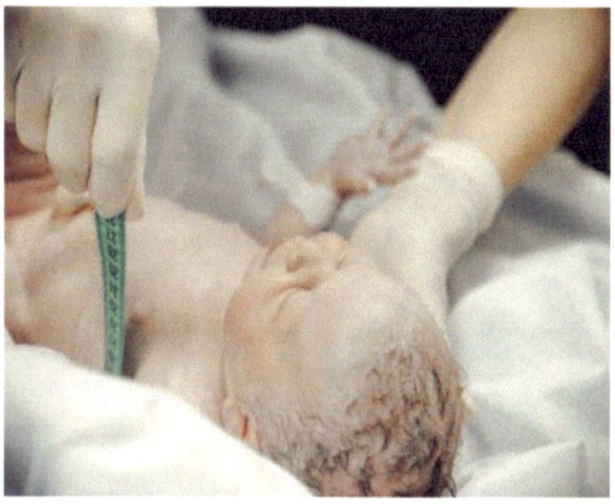

However, when health care workers provide expectant and/or new mothers with infant formula promotion materials they mistakably reduce an infant's likelihood of being breastfeed. Studies show mothers who receive discharge packages containing items useful for breastfeeding are more likely to breastfeed than mothers who receive discharge packages including free formula samples and coupons [18]. The sooner a mother opts out of breastfeeding, the more formula is purchased, which creates an incentive for formula companies to market infant formula to women even before giving birth which is usually when prenatal intention to breast or formula feed is established.

The practices of maternity hospitals regarding breastfeeding as well as the attitudes and information provided by healthcare workers regarding infant feeding largely influences infant feeding behaviors. Health providers and maternity facilities that disseminate information regarding the benefits of breastfeeding as well as provide useful breastfeeding resources have the potential to significantly increase breastfeeding prevalence [18]. In 1991, the WHO and UNICEF initiated the Baby-Friendly Hospital Initiative, with the goal of improving maternity facilities to better support and promote breastfeeding. A facility must follow the "Ten Steps to Successful Breastfeeding" (described in **Table 2** below) in order to be designated as a "Baby-friendly" facility [1] (**Table 3**).

1. Fund breastfeeding programs that will build advocacy and garner political support for breastfeeding.
2. Regulate the promotion of infant formula.
3. Enact legislation to protect the rights of breastfeeding women and advocate for paid maternity leave.
4. Provide breastfeeding support and maternity services, including lactation counseling and peer support programs.
5. Improve community support for breastfeeding and integrate the voices of mothers, spouses and their families into breastfeeding advocacy campaigns.
6. Develop systems to monitor and improve breastfeeding programs.
7. Disseminate accurate information on the value and significance of breastfeeding.

Table 2.
The World Health Assembly call to action to support breastfeeding [11].

1. Have a written breastfeeding policy that is communicated to all health care staff.
2. Train all health care staff in the skills necessary to implement this policy.
3. Inform all new mothers about the benefits of exclusive breastfeeding
4. Assist mothers in initiating breastfeeding within a half hour of an infant's birth
5. Show mothers how to breastfeed and how to maintain lactation, even if they are separated from their infants.
6. Do not give infants any food or drink other than breastmilk, unless supplemental food is medically necessary
7. Allow mothers and infants to room-in or stay in the same room at all times during their stay in the facility
8. Encourage breastfeeding on demand.
9. Do not give pacifiers or artificial nipples to breastfeeding infants.
10. Foster the establishment of breastfeeding support groups and refer mothers to them upon discharge from the hospital or birth center

Table 3.
Ten steps to successful breastfeeding [1].

3.4 Societal factors

3.4.1 Legislation

Policies that protect and support breastfeeding are necessary in order to enable a mother's decision to initiate and sustain breastfeeding. A majority of the approximate 1 million women who are employed full-time around the world do not benefit from supportive workplace policies regarding breastfeeding [2, 4]. The large prevalence and increase of women working outside the home is often cited for the low rates of breastfeeding indicating the necessity of workplace policies to support working mothers [7]. It is necessary that a woman has the time, space, privacy, and place to express milk in the workplace and in public areas [10]. Legislation in support of a women's choice to breastfeed can help overcome employment barriers and aid in the return of breastfeeding becoming the societal norm and standard feeding practice [10].

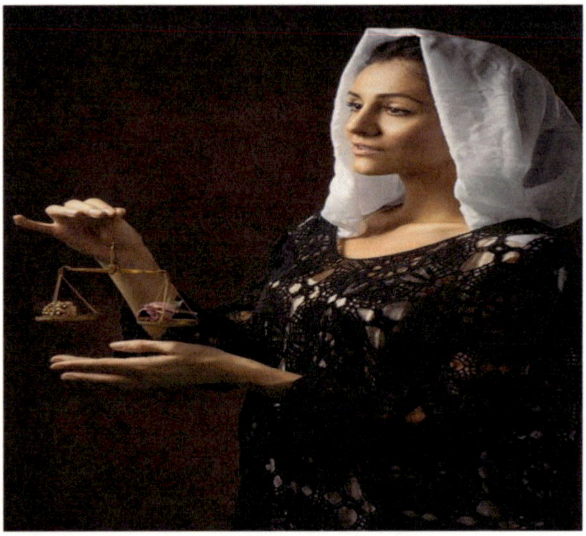

The lack of legislative accommodation in the workplace is a significant predictor of shorter duration of exclusive breastfeeding. Key workplace barriers include the lack of flexibility for milk expression in the work schedule, lack of accommodations such as a nursing room equipped to enable mothers to pump or store breastmilk, and concerns about employer or co-worker support [10]. Additional workplace barriers include the perception that breastfeeding may hinder a mothers' job performance, lack of privacy for expressing breast milk or for breastfeeding, and the inability to find a child care facility near the workplace, the high cost of day care, insurance regulations, employer building codes, and other rules that may limit infants and children in the workplace. Studies illustrate that supportive work site environments that provide a private place to express milk and access to a quality breast pump helps women to continue breastfeeding upon return to work [19].

Workplace policies such as paid breaks for expressing milk, the provision of lactation rooms, and public awareness of the breastfeeding policies, have the ability to improve the ability of mothers to sustain breastfeeding while working. Using data from 182 countries, Atabay and colleagues (2015) found the prevalence of exclusive breastfeeding among infants 6 months and younger was nearly 9 percentage points higher in countries with guaranteed paid breastfeeding work breaks compared to those without paid breaks [9]. Another study conducted in 2014, found 136 out of 176 countries, or approximately 71% of the world, provided mothers the right to take paid breaks during the workday in order to provide breastmilk for their child until 6 months following birth while four countries permitted shorter or unpaid breastfeeding breaks. However, 51 countries, the remaining 29% of the world, did not have policies that protected the right of mothers to breastfeed [9].

Further, research illustrates extended maternity leave is associated with higher prevalence of exclusive breastfeeding because women are able to continue breastfeeding without choosing between employment and providing breastmilk for her child. A report by the International Labor Organization found that in most developed countries 75–100% of pay was guaranteed for up to 16 weeks of maternity leave. In over 70 countries, employers are paid through social security systems in order to decrease cost burdens [20]. The United States does not have a universal policy that guarantees paid maternity leave and also has one of the lowest rates of breastfeeding and one of the highest rates of infant mortality among developed countries. A study examining 16 countries found maternity leave policies increase breastfeeding prevalence and prevent one to two neonatal deaths per 2000 live births [21]. In Norway, mothers can take up to 42 weeks of maternity leave with full pay or receive 80% pay for 52 weeks. More than 97% of Norwegian women initiate breastfeeding and 80% continue to do so until at least 3 months; this is largely different from the 79% of American women who initiate breastfeeding and the 41% who still exclusively breastfeed at 3 months [20, 22]. Other interventions implemented in Norway to encourage breastfeeding include the availability of breastfeeding informational material, training health workers to help mothers have positive breastfeeding experiences, and establishing support groups where mother are able collectively share breastfeeding experiences [22]. Norwegian mothers who are employed are entitled to 60- to 90-minute daily breaks and can even leave to breastfeed their infant or have their infant brought to work. Supportive policies workplace policies are needed in order to improve breastfeeding rates and achieve the maximum benefits breastfeeding can offer [20].

3.4.2 Infant formula marketing

Women entering the labor force and the promotion of large-scale infant formula brands have drastically altered infant feeding practices. The provision of free infant formula samples in maternity facilities and the promotion of breastmilk substitutes by the media and healthcare providers have been shown to reduce breastfeeding prevalence [23]. Research indicates the use of infant formula is twice as high among mothers who have viewed and recalled an infant formula advertisement compared to mothers who had not viewed the advertisements [23].

The media, including marketing and advertisements, influence social norms, which are the shared beliefs regarding the acceptable behaviors within a social group [23]. The media also influences the attitudes toward behaviors and tend to appeal to prevalent values and perceptions in order to generate views and boost profits. For example, in 1997, Tabitha Walrond, a young black mother, was convicted of negligent homicide after her 2-month old child died from malnutrition. The mother was unaware that her breast reduction surgery from years prior would result in an insufficient supply of breastmilk. Years later, Walrond's case was depicted on a popular TV show, "Chicago Hope," which depicted breastfeeding to be potentially fatal. However, the episode portrayed white and middle-class parents (a more "appealing" demographic) who were being criminally investigated following the death of a breastfed child as a result of malnutrition. Rather than illustrating the -Friendly Hospital Initiative as an effort to enable successful breastfeeding the episode suggested the initiative was forcing mothers to breastfeed leading to infant deaths as a result of malnourishment. Alarmingly, the episode was also found to be a ploy by pharmaceutical companies to inform the public of the risks associated with breastfeeding [24].

Infant formula advertisements also appeal to common maternal experiences and concerns often suggesting breastmilk substitutes have ingredients that improve infant intelligence, solve digestive issues, and even help infants sleep through the night. Such claims have not been substantiated by research. However, research has recognized the association of breastfeeding with higher intelligence and reduced risk of gastrointestinal illness among many other health benefits. Digestive issues such as colic are no less prevalent in formula fed than breastfed infants and formula fed infants have not been found to sleep more than breastfed infants. Hunger is one of many reasons infants cry, thusly, infant formula is not associated with a reduced response of infant crying [23].

Further, media is often driven by profits and audience appeals. The external pressures stemming from the aggressive marketing of infant formula and media messages regarding formula can affect a mother's intent to breastfeed and provide the most optimal form of nutrition to her child [25]. The excessive marketing of infant formula and inaccurate portrayal of breastfeeding can undermine the significance of breastfeeding by spreading biased information and diminishing a mother's confidence in her ability to breastfeed. Infant formula is often portrayed to be as good as breastfeeding and a viable solution to a convenient lifestyle for working mothers. The labels displayed on infant formula often include descriptions such as "gold standard" and images depicting happy infants. This type of labeling implies positive health and developmental benefits, while ignoring the potential economic and health consequences associated with formula feeding [23]. However, families of breastfed infants can experience economic advantages in addition to health benefits. Infant formula can cost over $1500 throughout an infant's first year of life, however, women who breastfeed avoid the substantial cost burden [10]. Breastfed infants also require less medical attention rendering decreased medical expenses and fewer missed days of work for parents. A study found that a group of formula-fed infants had accrued $68,000 in health care costs over a 6-month timeframe, while an equal number of breastfeeding babies accrued only $4000 of similar medical expenses [26]. Breastfeeding is also better for the environment because less waste is produced compared to the waste created by formula products and bottle supplies. The media can play an integral role in disseminating such accurate and positive messages regarding breastfeeding. Media campaigns that are short, tailored to the needs and values of the audience, and displayed through the appropriate channel (e.g., radio, television, social media) that reaches and appeals to the target audience are most successful.

However, formula companies tend to make unsubstantiated claims regarding breastmilk substitutes and use trusted healthcare workers to promote infant formula. The provision of free infant formula samples in maternity facilities and the promotion of breastmilk substitutes by the media and healthcare providers have also been shown to reduce breastfeeding prevalence [23]. Infant formula companies attract new consumers by providing free samples and information on breastmilk substitutes to expectant and new mothers through providers and hospital facilities. Physicians are usually the most undisputed consultant on infant health and nutrition, making them a prime vehicle for promoting infant formula. Formula companies give doctors free or discounted products in exchange for physicians recommending and encouraging their brand of infant formula to expectant and new mothers. Many hospitals provide new mothers with packages containing free infant formula and coupons upon hospital discharge [23].

The marketing tactics employed by formula companies sparked international disapproval based on the assertion formula marketing led to preventable infant deaths. The international opposition prompted the WHO and UNICEF to develop the International Code of Marketing of Breastmilk Substitutes. The Code prohibits the unethical marketing of infant formula as equal to or superior to breastmilk and restricts the promotion of infant formula by medical practices [18]. Distributing accurate, unbiased information regarding the benefits of and importance of breastfeeding through the media as well as healthcare workers is critical to improving breastfeeding prevalence and reducing the dispersion of false information and misperceptions regarding the significance of breastfeeding.

4. Conclusion

Breastfeeding is considered the single most effective solution to preventing deaths of children under the age of five globally [26]. Considering the substantial economic and health savings that breastfeeding alone provides, exclusive breastfeeding should be supported and promoted within families, communities, workplaces, and hospital facilities that provide care to mothers and their infants. Understanding and addressing the dynamic interplay between individual, interpersonal, community, organizational and societal factors, such as policies and legislation that impact breastfeeding rates and the health of infants is key to improving breastfeeding prevalence. Below is an example of evidence-informed approaches used to improve the prevalence of exclusive breastfeeding that can be adapted and applied in both developing and developed countries.

5. Key strategies employed to increase global exclusive breastfeeding prevalence

Increasing Breastfeeding Prevalence in Cambodia

Over the span of a decade, Cambodia's breastfeeding rates increased from 11% in 2000 to 74% by 2010. Implementing the following recommendations that were informed by evidence in Cambodia can accelerate the progress towards reaching exclusive breastfeeding targets. The key strategies employed in Cambodia to increase breastfeeding rates included:

- Recognizing breastfeeding as a key strategy to child-survival interventions;
- Including breastfeeding promotion in all infant and children initiatives;
- Regulating the marketing of infant and children products;
- Initiating a "Baby-Friendly Child Initiative" involving the Baby-friendly Hospital Initiative and establishing maternal peer support groups and counseling services to support breastfeeding;
- Disseminating breastfeeding information through appropriate channels including popular TV and radio shows as well as launching a national breastfeeding advocacy campaign with high political officials [17].

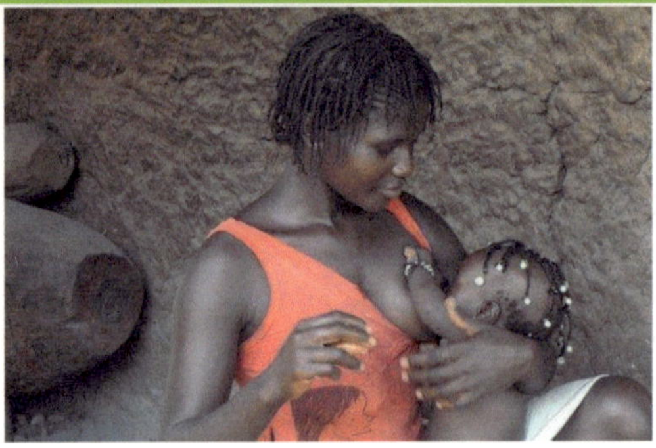

Conflict of interest

The author declares no conflict of interest.

Author details

Whitney N. Hamilton
Middle Georgia State University, Macon, United States

*Address all correspondence to: whitney.hamilton@mga.edu

References

[1] WHO/UNICEF. Global Nutrition Targets 2025: Breastfeeding Policy Brief [Internet]. 2014. Available from: https://www.who.int/nutrition/publications/globaltargets2025_policybrief_breastfeeding/en/ [Accessed: 04 December 2019]

[2] WHO/UNICEF. Nurturing the health and wealth of nations: The investment case for breastfeeding. Global Breastfeeding Collective - Executive Summary [Internet]. 2017. Available from: https://www.who.int/nutrition/publications/infantfeeding/global-bf-collective-investmentcase/en/ [Accessed: 04 December 2019]

[3] Victora CG, Bahl R, Barros AJ, Franca GV, Horton S, Krasevec J, et al. Breastfeeding in the 21st century: Epidemiology, mechanisms, and lifelong effect. Lancet. 2016;**387**(10017):475-490. DOI: 10.1016/s0140-6736(15)01024-7

[4] WHO/UNICEF. Tracking Progress for Breastfeeding Policies and Programmes [Internet]. 2017. Available from: https://www.who.int/nutrition/publications/infantfeeding/global-bf-scorecard-2017.pdf [Accessed: 08 December 2019]

[5] Breastfeeding: Achieving the new normal. The Lancet. 2016;**387**(10017):404. DOI: 10.1016/S0140-6736(16)00210-5

[6] Bentley ME, Dee DL, Jensen JL. Breastfeeding among low income, African-American women: Power, beliefs and decision making. The Journal of Nutrition. 2003;**133**(1):305S-309S. DOI: 10.1093/jn/133.1.305S

[7] Murtagh L, Moulton AD. Working mothers, breastfeeding, and the law. American Journal of Public Health. 2011;**101**(2):217-223. DOI: 10.2105/ajph.2009.185280

[8] Earle S. Factors affecting the initiation of breastfeeding: Implications for breastfeeding promotion. Health Promotion International. 2002;**17**(3):205-214 https://doi.org/10.1093/heapro/17.3.205

[9] Atabay E, Moreno G, Nandi A, Kranz G, Vincent I, Assi TM, et al. Facilitating working mothers' ability to breastfeed: Global trends in guaranteeing breastfeeding breaks at work, 1995-2014. Journal of Human Lactation. 2015;**31**(1):81-88. DOI: 10.1177/0890334414554806

[10] Office of the Surgeon, Centers for Disease Control and Prevention, & Office on Women's Health. Publications and reports of the surgeon general. In: The Surgeon General's Call to Action to Support Breastfeeding. Rockville (MD): Office of the Surgeon General (US); 2011

[11] WHO/UNICEF. Breastfeeding and gender equality. Breastfeeding Advocacy Brief [Internet]. 2019. Available from: https://www.unicef.org/nutrition/files/6._Advocacy_Brief_on_BF_and_Gender_Equality.pdf [Accessed: 04 December, 2019]

[12] Balogun OO, Dagvadorj A, Anigo KM, Ota E, Sasaki S. Factors influencing breastfeeding exclusivity during the first 6 months of life in developing countries: A quantitative and qualitative systematic review. Maternal & Child Nutrition. 2015;**11**:433-451. DOI: 10.1111/mcn.12180

[13] Reeta B. Breast feeding in developing countries: Is there a scope for improvement. Journal of Neonatal Biology. 2016;**5**(1):2-5. DOI: 10.4172/2167-0897.1000208

[14] Sparks PJ. Differences in breastfeeding initiation in the United States. Journal of Human Lactation. 2010;**26**(2):118-129. DOI: 10.1177/0890334409352854

[15] Maharlouei N, Pourhaghighi A, Shahraki HR, Zohoori D, Lankarani KB. Factors affecting exclusive breastfeeding, using adaptive LASSO regression. International Journal of Community Based Nursing & Midwifery. 2018;**6**(3):260-271

[16] James RS. Breastfeeding disparities in African American women. National Institute on Minority Health and Health Disparities [Internet]. 2017. Available from: https://nimhd.blogs.govdelivery.com/2017/08/08/breastfeeding-disparities-in-african-american-women/ [Accessed: 02 January 2020]

[17] Kimani-Murage EW, Wekesah F, Wanjohi M, Kyobutungi C, Ezeh AC, Musoke RN, et al. Factors affecting actualisation of the WHO breastfeeding recommendations in urban poor settings in Kenya. Maternal & Child Nutrition. 2015;**11**(3):314-332. DOI: 10.1111/mcn.12161

[18] Kaplan D, Graff K. Marketing breastfeeding- reversing corporate influence on infant feeding practices. Journal of Urban Health. 2008;**85**(4):486-504. DOI: 10.1007/s11524-008-9279-6

[19] Investing in Workplace Breastfeeding Programs. National Business Group on Health: Center for Prevention and Health Services [Internet]. 2009. Available from: https://www.businessgrouphealth.org/pub/?id=f2ffe4f0-2354-d714-5136-79a21e9327ed. [Accessed: 04 November 2019]

[20] Raju TN. Continued barriers for breast-feeding in public and the workplace. The Journal of Pediatrics. 2006;**148**(5):677-679.e671. DOI: 10.1016/j.jpeds.2005.12.034

[21] Stuebe AM, Michels KB, Willett WC, Manson JE, Rexrode K, Rich-Edwards JW. Duration of lactation and incidence of myocardial infarction in middle to late adulthood. American Journal of Obstetrics and Gynecology. 2009;**200**(2):138.e131-138.e138. DOI: 10.1016/j.ajog.2008.10.001

[22] Lubold AM. The effect of family policies and public health initiatives on breastfeeding initiation among 18 high-income countries: A qualitative comparative analysis research design. International Breastfeeding Journal. 2017;**12**(1):34. DOI: 10.1186/s13006-017-0122-0

[23] Piwoz E, Huffman S. The impact of marketing breast-milk substitutes on WHO-recommended breastfeeding practices. Food and Nutrition Bulletin. 2015;**36**(4):373-386. DOI: 10.1177/0379572115602174

[24] Brown J, Peuchard SR. Media and breastfeeding: Friend or foe. International Breastfeeding Journal. 2008;**3**(15):1-3. DOI: 10.1186/1746-4358-3-15

[25] Baker P, Smith J, Salmon L, Friel S, Kent G, Iellamo A, et al. Global trends and patterns of commercial milk-based formula sales: Is an unprecedented infant and young child feeding transition underway? Public Health Nutrition. 2016;**19**(14):2540-2550. DOI: 10.1017/S1368980016001117

[26] Hahn-Holbrook J, Schetter CD, Haselton M. Breastfeeding and maternal mental and physical health. Reproductive Health. 2012:414-438

Section 3

Breast Feeding: Ocular and Hematopoietic Effects

Chapter 4

Relationship between Ocular Morbidity and Infant Nutrition

Erdinc Bozkurt and Hayrunisa Bekis Bozkurt

Abstract

The nutrition of the constantly growing and developing infant even after birth has an undeniable contribution to the development of eyes, which can be considered as the extension of the brain. Therefore, the elucidation of these physiological developments is valuable in terms of preventing pathological conditions. During the first six months of an infant's life, nutrition is provided through breast milk or infant formula, and after the sixth month, there is a transition to additional food. Breast milk is, thus, considered as 'miracle food', with a growing body of research being undertaken to investigate its relationship with orbital diseases and reporting that breast milk reduces ocular morbidity. Breast milk is an accessible, economical and important nutrition source for eye development and infant health. The developments in recent years have resulted in the content of formula being closer to that of breast milk, which can positively affect the neurovisional development of babies that cannot be fed with breast milk.

Keywords: breastfeeding, formula, infant, visual development, refractive disorders, retinal disease

1. Nutrition in the first year of life and orbital development

Orbital development begins in fourth to sixth weeks of the intrauterine period. The eye develops from the surface ectoderm, neural ectoderm, and mesoderm. The optic nerve is also seen as an extension of the brain [1]. There is a significant relationship between the mother's diet during pregnancy and the orbital development of the infant. In recent years, the concept of the "first 1000" days emerged to refer to the process during pregnancy and the first two years after birth. The first 1000 days play a key role in many stages of life [2], and this period is also important in terms of healthy eye development and the prevention of orbital diseases, comorbid conditions, and complications.

The mother's diet during pregnancy is very valuable in terms of providing essential fatty acids and amino acids, which are necessary for the development of the orbital tissues of the infant. Studies have shown this developmental process is positively affected by a diet rich in phospholipids (PL), phosphatidylcholine (PC), phosphatidylethanolamine (PE), N-acylphosphatidylethanolamine (NAPE), phosphatidylinositol (PI), and phosphatidylserine (PS) [3]. Similarly, the mother's malnutrition during breastfeeding in the first year after birth negatively affects the orbital and brain development of the infant. In the complex process of orbital and visual development, tissues and cells need many minerals, vitamins and nutrients to continue their functions [4]. For example, in this process, vitamin A plays a vital role for photoreceptors, vitamin C is important for the development of the aqueous humor, and fatty acids are essential for the development of the optic nerve and myelin sheath [5]. In recent years, with the development of technology, premature infants now live longer, and the nutrition and supportive treatments for premature newborns have become even more important. In these infants, retinopathy of prematurity (ROP), which can cause blindness when not treated early, is seen very often due to hyperoxia, long stay in mechanical ventilation, infection, prematurity, low birth weight, and low-calorie maternal diet [6]. A diet rich in vitamins A and E, and longer duration of breastfeeding decreases the requirement of surgery to treat ROP [7, 8].

The nutrition of the constantly growing and developing infant even after birth has an undeniable contribution to the development of eyes, which can be considered as the extension of the brain. Therefore, the elucidation of these physiological developments is valuable in terms of preventing pathological conditions [9]. During the first six months of an infant's life, nutrition is provided through breast milk or infant formula, and after the sixth month, there is a transition to additional food. In this chapter, we discuss breast milk, infant formula, and their relationship with ocular morbidity.

2. Breast milk: the best nutrition for orbital development

After the baby is born, breastfeeding especially in the first six months is considered as a fundamental right by WHO and necessary actions are taken to ensure this for every child [10]. Breast milk is the most suitable food for a newborn in terms of the balance of nutrients it contains [11]. Studies have shown that breast milk protects the infant against many diseases, malignancies, obesity, and malnutrition [12]. Degeneration occurs in retinal ganglion cells and photoreceptors, especially when the infant's diet is deficient in taurine found at high levels in breast milk [13]. Many bioactive compounds, such as α-lactalbumin, lactoferrin and immunoglobulins, which have antioxidant properties, are known to be important for brain and orbital development, as well as immunomodulatory functions [14]. Being rich in glial cell-line derived neurotrophic factor (GDNF) and oligosaccharides, breast milk acts as an important stimulator for healthy development [15]. The presence of many growth factors and the importance of the baby being in proper osmolarity and balance for the full development of the intestines and kidneys further increase the value of breast milk [16]. Breast milk is, thus, considered as 'miracle food', with a growing body of research being undertaken to investigate its relationship with orbital diseases and reporting that breast milk reduces ocular morbidity [17].

3. New formulas enriched with vitamin and minerals

In circumstances where breast milk is insufficient or contraindicated, the use of formula approaching breast milk in terms of content has increased in recent years. Infant formula can be divided into three groups as soy-based, cow milk-based and hypoallergic or amino acid-based special foods produced for special conditions, such as metabolic diseases [18]. However, there have been discussions of safety for formula in terms of infant health since its first use [19]. Due to the high levels of renal solute load of the foods used in the first year of life, infant formula still lags behind breast milk, and there are only limited scientific studies on the relationship between infant formula and highly critical molecules for brain and eye development, . Considering the positive impact of breast milk on the immune system, the food given to the infant in case of breast milk deficiency or contraindication should be "closest" to breast milk [20]. With the latest technologies, the enrichment of formula foods with prebiotics, probiotics, oligosaccharides, and various vitamins and minerals has made significant contributions to infant nutrition [21]. In particular, molecules which take part in the development of visual functions, such as docosahexaenoic acid (DHA), vitamin A, and vitamin E have started to be added to infant formula. In a study on baby rhesus monkeys, it was observed that formula enriched with carotenoid increased the amount of lutein in the brain and tissues and positively affected their development, but not to the extent of the positive effect of breast milk [22].

A healthy and balanced nutrition in childhood is very important for not only growth and development and but also prevention of diseases. In terms of eye health, it is important to ensure that the infant receives age-appropriate nutrition with breast milk and foods close to breast milk in content and quality, which will protect her/him against malnutrition and obesity and an adequate intake of vitamins and minerals.

4. Breastfeeding and ocular disease

4.1 Breastfeeding and visual development

Breast milk contains an average of 1.1% protein, 4.2% fat, and 7.0% carbohydrates, and is a miraculous nutrient in which every 100 g contains 72 kcal energy [23]. Breast milk also has vitamins E and C, as well as enzymes, such as superoxide dismutase, catalase, and glutathione peroxidase with strong antioxidant properties. In this way, it protects the infant from eye damage that may be caused by oxidative stress [24]. Generally, breast milk has been found to be inadequate in certain vitamins and minerals, such as vitamin D, iodine, iron, and vitamin K. Since the deficiency of these vitamins and minerals can affect the infant systematically, going beyond eye diseases, they are usually added to the infant's diet as supplements [25].

Breast milk supports the infant's growth and development through its content of long-chain polyunsaturated essential fatty acids, such as arachidonic acid, long chain polyunsaturated fatty acids (LC-PUFAs) (20: 4n-6) and DHA (22: 6n-3), linoleic (LA; 18: 2n-6) and alpha-linolenic (18: 3n-3) acid [26]. DHA and arachidonic acid (AA) in the membrane lipids of the brain and retina are critical for visual and neuronal functions. Taking these substances with diet in the first year of life is important for the visual development of infants [27].

The retina (and the crystalline lens to a lesser extent) has reduced light-sourced oxidative damage by vitamin E and C, and carotenoids (lutein and zeaxanthin), which are intensely present in the macular region. Vitamins E and C and lutein cannot be synthesized by the infant, and therefore should be taken in through the diet [28]. Dietary carotenoid, lutein and zeoxanthin are known to be protective against some eye diseases, such as macular degenerations [29]. It was observed that the serum lutein level of infants fed with breast milk was higher than that of infants fed with formula [30]. This indicates that infants fed with breast milk may be resistant to many eye diseases caused by oxidative damage due to its higher antioxidant levels than formula. Vitamin A is an important vitamin used by photoreceptors in visual physiology. Adequate intake of vitamin A, which is found in breast milk and formula foods, has been shown to reduce the severity of ROP through vascular endothelial growth factor (VEGF-A). In addition, preterm infants fed with breast milk have higher serum insulin-like growth factor-1 (IGF-1) levels than those who feed with formula [31]. A high IGF-1 level decreases the severity of ROP by ensuring the normal development of retinal vascularization [32].

4.2 Refractive disorders and breastfeeding

Refractive disorders (error) represent a mismatch between the focal and axial lengths of the eye. The 10th revision of the International Classification of Diseases, defines this disorder as blurring in vision as a result of a defect in focusing light on the retina [33]. At birth, the average cycloplegic refractive error for the infant usually ranges from ±1.50 dioptre (D) to ±2.50 D, with standard deviations from +1.00 to +2.50 D [34]. At the age of six to 72 months, the eyes undergo a process of emmetropization in which the average refractive error decreases in both myopic and hypermetropic infants [35].

Refractive disorders are the most common cause of visual impairment and the second most common cause of treatable visual deficiency [36]. The frequency of refractive disorders may vary according to ethnicity, age, and the development level of the country [37]. According to a study carried out in the USA in 2015, the frequency of visual impairment in children between the ages of three and five is estimated to be around 1.5%, which is expected to increase in the near future [38]. Among the most important etiological causes of refractive disorders are genetics and gene-environment interactions [39–41]. In addition, nutrition is considered to have an impact on refractive disorder and orbital health. It is stated that the prevalence of refractive disorders, such as ametropia, anisometropia and astigmatism is high, especially in African societies exposed to malnutrition [37].

Recently, the effect of breast milk intake, which is the most important source of infant nutrition, on refractive disorders has been investigated. It is thought that breastfeeding is important for visual development and orbital growth during the infantile period [42]. In one of these studies, it was shown that breast milk-fed children of mothers with a DHA-rich diet had better stereoscopic vision than the formula-fed children [43].

Refractive disorders can be basically classified as myopia, hyperopia, and astigmatism. Myopia is one of the most common visual impairments and has become an important public health problem due to its increasing prevalence in recent years. While the prevalence of ametropia, anisometropia, and astigmatism is high in Africa, the frequency of myopia is low in developing countries while it is higher in developed societies, such as the United States of America (USA) and the United Kingdom (UK) [44]. This is not a surprising finding considering that myopia is associated with reading and using technological devices, which require looking at objects closely.

In a study carried out in Singapore, high levels of unsaturated fatty acids and cholesterol intake were associated with longer AL, although they could not be directly associated with myopia [45]. In another study undertaken by Liu et al. in China, it was found that feeding the infant with breast milk for the first six months was associated with hyperopic spherical equivalent refraction (SER) and less myopia and was not related to AL [46]. However, in the study of Growing Up in Singapore Towards Healthy Outcomes (GUSTO), infant feeding at the sixth, ninth and 12th months did not affect the myopia levels at the age of 3.5 years [47].

There are also many studies suggesting that breastfeeding has no effect on myopia. In a study on strabismus, amblyopia and refractive disorder (STARS) conducted with 797 children in Singapore, 65.4% of the sample were myopic, of which 8.5% were breastfed. In that study, it was stated that there was no relationship between breast milk and myopia [48]. In another study supporting the STARS study, it was reported that breast milk had no effect on myopia [49]. In a study which included 311 children in Iran (grades 1–5), the rate of breastfeeding for more than six months was 85% while the frequency of myopia (SE of at least −0.50 D) was 5.2%. It was stated that the breastfeeding of the infant for the first six months had no significant effect on vision level or refractive error [50]. A study undertaken in the UK suggested that other factors, such as parental education status, gender, maternal age, and order of birth were more important for visual development and myopia in early life than the type of infant feeding [49]. The existence of different opinions and findings on this subject indicates that further detailed studies are needed.

Another refractive defect is hypermetropia, which occurs due to either the AL of the eye being shorter than normal or refractive structures such as cornea and lens having less refractive power than normal [51]. In a study investigating the relationship between hyperopia and breastfeeding, it was stated that breastfeeding resulted in a significantly high rate of hyperopia. This increased incidence of hyperopia was associated with various reasons, such as ethnicity, presence of refractive disorder, ethnic and sociocultural structure, and content of the mother's milk [52]. Bozkurt et al. stated that although breastfeeding leads to a hyperopic shift, it has no effect on SER [53].

Another refractive disorder, astigmatism, occurs as a result of the refractive parts of the eye (cornea and lens) not producing an equal amount of refraction on each meridian, leading to images not being focused on a point on the fovea. Generally, the breaking force of the vertical axis of the anterior aspect of the cornea is 0.5 D more than its horizontal axis. This condition, known as physiological astigmatism, is reduced to zero by the cornea posterior face and lens. Lenticular (lens-dependent) astigmatism is rarer. The image of an object being in the form of two separate lines, 90° perpendicular to each other in two planes, is called regular astigmatism, which is the most common type of astigmatism in the clinic [54]. The prevalence of astigmatism can be seen in different countries at different frequencies. While this rate is 2.2% in Nepal, it reaches 82.2% in Singapore [55, 56]. Since there is only limited information in the literature investigating the relationship between breastfeeding and astigmatism, we consider that there is not yet enough data to support the presence of such relationship.

4.3 Breastfeeding and retinal disease

The retina, which is considered an extension of the brain, has two major layers as the outer retinal pigment epithelium and the inner neurosensory layer. The neurosensory layer is formed by a photoreceptor layer, bipolar ganglion, amacrine and horizontal cells, and support cells similar to neuroglia [57]. When the pathologies that may occur with inflammation, trauma, autoimmune or epigenetic mechanisms in each layer are examined, it is seen that they are associated with the deficiency of vitamins and minerals [58, 59].

In addition to except vitamins K and D, breast milk is very rich in other vitamins and minerals that are indispensable elements of a healthy and balanced nutrition. Furthermore, polyunsaturated fatty acids and antioxidants in breast milk play an important role in the development of the eye and neuronal structure in the first months of life [48]. The leading chemical structures that contribute to the development of the brain and retina in breast milk are LA, α-LA, AA, and DHA [60], which are commonly called LC-PUFAs. In animal experiments, DHA deficiency has been shown to cause the impairment of neuronal and retinal functions [61]. It has also been reported that the photoreceptor external segments of monkeys fed with a diet devoid of taurine amino acid are degenerated, and taurine is abundantly found in breast milk [62].

Another important molecule, phosphatidylcholine, is essential for the synthesis of phospholipids, DNA methylation, and the neurodevelopmental process of infants. In an animal experiment study conducted by Surzenko et al., it was shown that a low choline diet during pregnancy affected the retinal development and function in the fetus, and choline provided differentiation and proliferation in retinal progenitor cells [63]. Infants received enough choline and LC-PUFAs from breast milk, which are very important for the brain, retinal and neurovisional development. In another study, it was emphasized that formula foods containing choline and LC-PUFAs were required for growth and development in non-breastfed infants [64].

The thickness of the retinal nerve fiber layer (RNFL) can offer an idea about retinal structures in the early period. Conditions occurring in the retinal layers, such as edema and atrophy can be objectively evaluated using optical coherence tomography. In a study undertaken by Bozkurt et al., stated that the retinal nerve fiber layer was thicker in formula-fed children, than breast-fed infant, which might be related to the content of formula. However, a definitive conclusion could not be reached as to whether the thickening of RNFL in formula-fed infants was a healthy neurotrophy or an adaptive change [53].

Another important eye disease associated with infant nutrition is ROP, which occurs in preterm babies (birth week <37) with an immature retinal structure and not fully developed retinal vasculature. Today, ROP is considered as the most important cause of preventable blindness in childhood in developed and developing countries all over the world [65]. There are many studies showing the relationship between ROP and breast milk intake. For example, Okamoto et al. reported that the content of breast milk could reduce ROP severity and the ingredients in breast milk could protect premature infants from blindness [66]. In another study, Hylander et al. found that antioxidant substances, such as inositol, vitamin E, and beta carotene in breast milk prevented ROP development, and formula-fed infants had a higher ROP frequency than breast-fed infants, especially due to the absence of inositol in standard formula [67]. In another study supporting this study, the supplementation of infant diet with inositol was shown to reduce the incidence of ROP [68]. ROP is the most serious retinal disease that causes the deficiency of vision in the neonatal period, secondary to retinal detachment. According to the literature, breast milk intake should be encouraged to reduce the harm caused by ROP [66, 67].

In conclusion, breast milk is an accessible, economical and important nutrition source for eye development and infant health. The developments in recent years have resulted in the content of formula being closer to that of breast milk, which can positively affect the neurovisional development of babies that cannot be fed with breast milk.

Author details

Erdinc Bozkurt[1*] and Hayrunisa Bekis Bozkurt[2]

1 Department of Ophthalmology, Kafkas University, Faculty of Medicine, Kars, Turkey

2 Department of Pediatrics, Kafkas University, Faculty of Medicine, Kars, Turkey

*Address all correspondence to: drerdincbozkurt@hotmail.com

References

[1] Lutty GA, DS ML. Development of the hyaloid, choroidal and retinal vasculatures in the fetal human eye. Progress in Retinal and Eye Research. 2018;**62**:58-76

[2] Cusick SE, Georgieff MK. The role of nutrition in brain development: The golden opportunity of the "first 1000 days". The Journal of Pediatrics. 2016;**175**:16-21

[3] Destaillats F, Bezelgues J-B, Dionisi F, Cruz-Hernandez C. Long-chain polyunsaturated fatty acids (lc-pufa) in maternal nutrition during pregnancy and lactation [Google Patents]; 2011

[4] Miesfeld JB, Brown NL. Eye organogenesis: A hierarchical view of ocular development. Current Topics in Developmental Biology. 2019;**132**:351-393

[5] McLaren DS. Malnutrition and the eye. New York: Academic Press; 2014. pp. 172-179, 213-214

[6] Hellström A, Smith LE, Dammann OJ. Retinopathy of prematurity. Lancet. 2013;**382**(9902):1445-1457

[7] Porcelli PJ, Weaver RG Jr. The influence of early postnatal nutrition on retinopathy of prematurity in extremely low birth weight infants. Early Human Development. 2010;**86**(6):391-396

[8] Sjöström ES, Lundgren P, Öhlund I, Holmström G, Hellström A, Domellöf MJ, et al. Low energy intake during the first 4 weeks of life increases the risk for severe retinopathy of prematurity in extremely preterm infants. BMJ Journals. 2016;**101**(2):F108-FF13

[9] Brown NAP, Bron AJ, Harding JJ, Dewar HM. Nutrition supplements and the eye. Eye. 1998;**12**(1):127-133

[10] Grummer-Strawn LM, Zehner E, Stahlhofer M, Lutter C, Clark D, Sterken E, et al. New World Health Organization guidance helps protect breastfeeding as a human right. Maternal & Child Nutrition. 2017;**13**(4):e12491

[11] Eidelman AI, Schanler RJ. Section on Breastfeeding. Breastfeeding and the Use of Human Milk. Pediatrics. 2012;**129**(3)

[12] Victora CG, Bahl R, Barros AJ, França GV, Horton S, Krasevec J, et al. Breastfeeding in the 21st century: Epidemiology, mechanisms, and lifelong effect. The Lancet. 2016;**387**(10017):475-490

[13] Gaucher D, Arnault E, Husson Z, Froger N, Dubus E, Gondouin P, et al. Taurine deficiency damages retinal neurones: Cone photoreceptors and retinal ganglion cells. Amino Acids. 2012;**43**(5):1979-1993

[14] Ballard O, Morrow AL. Human milk composition: Nutrients and bioactive factors. Pediatric Clinics. 2013;**60**(1):49-74

[15] Rodrigues D, Li A, Nair D, Blennerhassett MJ. Glial cell line-derived neurotrophic factor is a key neurotrophin in the postnatal enteric nervous system. Neurogastroenterology and Motility. 2011;**23**(2):e44-e56

[16] Kobata R, Tsukahara H, Ohshima Y, Ohta N, Tokuriki S, Tamura S, et al. High levels of growth factors in human breast milk. Early Human Development. 2008;**84**(1):67-69

[17] Aksoy A, Ozdemir M, Aslan L, Aslankurt M, Gul O. Effect of breast feeding on ocular morbidity. Medical Science Monitor. 2014;**20**:24

[18] Martin CR, Ling P-R, Blackburn GL. Review of infant feeding: Key features

of breast milk and infant formula. Nutrients. 2016;**8**(5):279

[19] Baker RD. Infant formula safety. Pediatrics. 2002;**110**(4):833-835

[20] Zou L, Pande G, Akoh CC. Infant formula fat analogs and human milk fat: New focus on infant developmental needs. Annual Review of Food Science and Technology. 2016;**7**:139-165

[21] Papagaroufalis K, Fotiou A, Egli D, Tran L-A, Steenhout P. A randomized double blind controlled safety trial evaluating d-lactic acid production in healthy infants Fed a lactobacillus reuteri-containing formula. Nutrition and Metabolic Insights. 2014;**7**:NMI-S14113

[22] Jeon S, Ranard KM, Neuringer M, Johnson EE, Renner L, Kuchan MJ, et al. Lutein is differentially deposited across brain regions following formula or breast feeding of infant rhesus macaques. The Journal of Nutrition. 2018;**148**(1):31-39

[23] Hanson LÅ, Korotkova M, Telemo E. Breast-feeding, infant formulas, and the immune system. Annals of Allergy, Asthma & Immunology. 2003;**90**(6):59-63

[24] Tsopmo A, Friel JK. Human milk has anti-oxidant properties to protect premature infants. Current Pediatric Reviews. 2007;**3**(1):45-51

[25] Erick M. Breast milk is conditionally perfect. Medical Hypotheses. 2018;**111**:82-89

[26] Yuhas R, Pramuk K, Lien EL. Human milk fatty acid composition from nine countries varies most in DHA. Lipids. 2006;**41**(9):851-858

[27] Birch EE, Castaneda YS, Wheaton DH, Birch DG, Uauy RD, Hoffman DR. Visual maturation of term infants fed long-chain polyunsaturated fatty acid-supplemented or control formula for 12 mo. The American Journal of Clinical Nutrition. 2005;**81**(4):871-879

[28] JP SG, Chew EY, Clemons TE, Ferris FL 3rd, Gensler G, et al. The relationship of dietary carotenoid and vitamin A, E, and C intake with age-related macular degeneration in a case-control study: AREDS Report No. 22. Archives of Ophthalmology. 2007;**125**(9):1225-1232

[29] Lien EL, Hammond BR. Nutritional influences on visual development and function. Progress in Retinal and Eye Research. 2011;**30**(3):188-203

[30] Handelman GJ, Dratz EA, Reay CC, van Kuijk JG. Carotenoids in the human macula and whole retina. Investigative Ophthalmology & Visual Science. 1988;**29**(6):850-855

[31] Alzaree FA, AbuShady MM, Atti MA, Fathy GA, Galal EM, Ali A, et al. Effect of early breast milk nutrition on serum insulin-like growth factor-1 in preterm infants. Open Access Macedonian Journal of Medical Sciences. 2019;**7**(1):77-81

[32] Hard AL, Smith LE, Hellstrom A. Nutrition, insulin-like growth factor-1 and retinopathy of prematurity. Seminars in Fetal & Neonatal Medicine. 2013;**18**(3):136-142

[33] WHO. International statistical classification of diseases, injuries and causes of death, tenth revision. Geneva, 1993. In: Quoted from Vision 2020 the Right to Sight Global Initiative for the Elimination of Avoidable Blindness: Action Plan 2006-2011. 2016

[34] Wood IC, Hodi S, Morgan L. Longitudinal change of refractive error in infants during the first year of life. Eye (London, England). 1995;**9**(Pt 5): 551-557

[35] Saunders KJ, Woodhouse JM, Westall CA. Emmetropisation in human infancy: Rate of change is related to initial refractive error. Vision Research. 1995;**35**(9):1325-1328

[36] Murthy GV, Gupta SK, Ellwein LB, Munoz SR, Pokharel GP, Sanga L, et al. Refractive error in children in an urban population in New Delhi. Investigative Ophthalmology & Visual Science. 2002;**43**(3):623-631

[37] Miller D, Atebara N, Fellenz M, Rosenthal P, Schechter R, West CJB, et al. Section 3: Optics, refraction, and contact lenses. In: Basic and Clinical Science Course. San Francisco: American Academy of Ophthalmology; 2004. p. 221

[38] Varma R, Tarczy-Hornoch K, Jiang X. Visual impairment in preschool children in the United States: Demographic and geographic variations from 2015 to 2060. JAMA Ophthalmology. 2017;**135**(6):610-616

[39] Saw SM, Chua WH, Hong CY, Wu HM, Chan WY, Chia KS, et al. Nearwork in early-onset myopia. Investigative Ophthalmology & Visual Science. 2002;**43**(2):332-339

[40] Seet B, Wong TY, Tan DT, Saw SM, Balakrishnan V, Lee LK, et al. Myopia in Singapore: Taking a public health approach. The British Journal of Ophthalmology. 2001;**85**(5):521-526

[41] Morgan I, Rose K. How genetic is school myopia? Progress in Retinal and Eye Research. 2005;**24**(1):1-38

[42] Heller CD, O'Shea M, Yao Q, Langer J, Ehrenkranz RA, Phelps DL, et al. Human milk intake and retinopathy of prematurity in extremely low birth weight infants. Pediatrics. 2007;**120**(1):1-9

[43] Williams C, Birch EE, Emmett PM, Northstone K. Stereoacuity at age 3.5 y in children born full-term is associated with prenatal and postnatal dietary factors: A report from a population-based cohort study. The American Journal of Clinical Nutrition. 2001;**73**(2):316-322

[44] Morgan IG, Ohno-Matsui K, Saw SM. Myopia. Lancet. 2012;**379**(9827):1739-1748

[45] Lim LS, Gazzard G, Low Y-L, Choo R, Tan DT, Tong L, et al. Dietary factors, myopia, and axial dimensions in children. Ophthalmology. 2010;**117, 5**:993-997

[46] Liu S, Ye S, Wang Q, Cao Y, Zhang X. Breastfeeding and myopia: A cross-sectional study of children aged 6-12 years in Tianjin, China. Scientific Reports. 2018;**8**(1):10025

[47] Chua SYL, Sabanayagam C, Tan CS, Lim LS, Toh JY, Chong YS, et al. Diet and risk of myopia in three-year-old Singapore children: The GUSTO cohort. Clinical and Experimental Optometry. 2018;**101**(5):692-699

[48] Chong Y-S, Liang Y, Tan D, Gazzard G, Stone RA, Saw S-M. Association between breastfeeding and likelihood of myopia in children. JAMA. 2005;**293**(24):2999-3002

[49] Rudnicka AR, Owen CG, Richards M, Wadsworth ME, Strachan DP. Effect of breastfeeding and sociodemographic factors on visual outcome in childhood and adolescence. The American Journal of Clinical Nutrition. 2008;**87**(5):1392-1399

[50] Shirzadeh E, Kooshki A, Mohammadi M. The relationship between breastfeeding and measurements of refraction and visual acuity in primary school children. Breastfeeding Medicine. 2016;**11**:235-238

[51] Flitcroft DI. Emmetropisation and the aetiology of refractive errors. Eye (London, England). 2014;**28**(2):169-179

[52] Sham WK, Dirani M, Chong YS, Hornbeak DM, Gazzard G, Li J, et al. Breastfeeding and association with refractive error in young Singapore Chinese children. Eye (London, England). 2010;**24**(5):875-880

[53] Bozkurt E, Bozkurt HB, Ucer MB. Comparative effect of feeding human milk as opposed to formula on visual function and ocular anatomy. Breastfeeding Medicine. 2019;**14**(7):493-498

[54] Grzybowski A, Kanclerz P. Beginnings of astigmatism understanding and management in the 19th century. Eye & Contact Lens. 2018;**44**(Suppl 1):S22-Ss9

[55] Pokharel GP, Negrel AD, Munoz SR, Ellwein LB. Refractive error study in children: Results from Mechi zone. Nepalese Journal of Ophthalmology. 2000;**129**(4):436-444

[56] Woo WW, Lim KA, Yang H, Lim XY, Liew F, Lee YS, et al. Refractive errors in medical students in Singapore. Singapore Medical Journal. 2004;**45**(10):470-474

[57] Burns SA, Elsner AE, Sapoznik KA, Warner RL, Gast TJ. Adaptive optics imaging of the human retina. Progress in Retinal and Eye Research. 2019;**68**:1-30

[58] Evans JR, Lawrenson JG. Antioxidant vitamin and mineral supplements for slowing the progression of age-related macular degeneration. The Cochrane Database of Systematic Reviews. 2017;7:CD000254

[59] Zhao Y, Feng K, Liu R, Pan J, Zhang L, Lu X. Vitamins and mineral supplements for retinitis pigmentosa. Journal of Ophthalmology. 2019;**2019**

[60] Innis SM. Impact of maternal diet on human milk composition and neurological development of infants. The American Journal of Clinical Nutrition. 2014;**99**(3):734S-741S

[61] Jeffrey BG, Mitchell DC, Hibbeln JR, Gibson RA, Chedester AL, Salem N Jr. Visual acuity and retinal function in infant monkeys fed long-chain PUFA. Lipids. 2002;**37**(9):839-848

[62] Liu A, Terry R, Lin Y, Nelson K, Bernstein PS. Comprehensive and sensitive quantification of long-chain and very long-chain polyunsaturated fatty acids in small samples of human and mouse retina. Journal of Chromatography. A. 2013;**1307**:191-200

[63] Surzenko N, Trujillo-González I, Zeisel SH. Low intake of choline during pregnancy leads to aberrant retinal architecture and poor visual function in the offspring. The FASEB Journal. 2016;**30**(1_supplement):679.9

[64] Mun JG, Legette LL, Ikonte CJ, Mitmesser SH. Choline and DHA in maternal and infant nutrition: Synergistic implications in brain and eye health. Nutrients. 2019;**11**(5)

[65] Quimson SK. Retinopathy of prematurity: Pathogenesis and current treatment options. Neonatal Network. 2015;**34**(5):284-287

[66] Okamoto T, Shirai M, Kokubo M, Takahashi S, Kajino M, Takase M, et al. Human milk reduces the risk of retinal detachment in extremely low-birthweight infants. Pediatrics International. 2007;**49**(6):894-897

[67] Hylander MA, Strobino DM, Pezzullo JC, Dhanireddy R. Association of human milk feedings with a reduction in retinopathy of prematurity among very low birthweight infants. Journal of Perinatology. 2001;**21**(6):356-362

[68] Hallman M, Bry K, Hoppu K, Lappi M, Pohjavuori M. Inositol supplementation in premature infants with respiratory distress syndrome. The New England Journal of Medicine. 1992;**326**(19):1233-1239

Chapter 5

Caseins as Regulators of Hematopoiesis

Edgar Ledesma-Martinez, Vanihamin Domínguez-Meléndez, Itzen Aguiñiga-Sánchez and Edelmiro Santiago-Osorio

Abstract

The main physiological role of casein, the main protein component in the milk, is to be a source of amino acids that are required for the growth of the neonate; therefore, casein is considered a highly nutritious protein. Over time, it has been revealed that casein is a protein whose physiological importance reaches levels far superior to the food field, having a wide array of biological activities including antimicrobial activities, facilitating absorption of nutrients, as well as acting as a growth factor and an immune stimulant. Here we analyze how caseins can exert numerous hematopoietic and immunomodulatory actions, their role in granulopoiesis, monocytopoiesis, and lymphopoiesis from the early stages of postnatal development seemingly throughout life, and we wonder if casein could be useful to fight pathogens resistant to antibiotics, inducing a strong immune response in immunosuppressed patients, or even be a prophylactic strategy to prevent infections.

Keywords: granulopoiesis, monocytopoiesis, lymphopoiesis, milk proteins, sodium caseinate

1. Introduction

Hematopoiesis is a process that includes the formation, maturation, and differentiation of blood cells. These cells have a relatively short life in circulation, so blood is a tissue with a high rate of renewal. The production of hematopoietic cells depends on a highly specialized bone marrow microenvironment, which regulates the quiescence, differentiation, and self-renewal of a rare population of multipotent cells known as hematopoietic stem cells (HSCs) and hematopoietic progenitor cells (HPCs), which give rise to all hematopoietic cell lineages [1].

The hematopoietic system plays numerous essential roles in human health and disease. Failure to maintain homeostasis in the blood system results in a range of human diseases, including anemia, hemophilia, immunodeficiency, allergies, leukemia, and lymphoma [2].

Studies in the past have consistently demonstrated that diet and nutritional status can significantly alter organismal physiology [3]. Thus, Kornberg et al. demonstrated over 60 years ago that amino acids were required for granulocyte and erythrocyte production; now, it is evident that disruption of dietary and metabolic factors [4], such as inadequate or imbalanced intake of macronutrients (carbohydrates, proteins, and fats) and micronutrients (vitamins and minerals), also known as "malnutrition," alters hematopoiesis and is generally associated with health risk markers [3]. In this sense, the organismal diet has emerged as an important regulator of adult HSC function [5].

Of the different types of malnutrition, protein restriction results from insufficient protein ingestion that can modify physiological responses and induce cellular disturbances, especially in tissues with a high rate of cellular renewal and proliferation, such as hematopoietic tissue; such process requires a large supply of nutrients as well as an organized structure for proliferation [6]. Protein malnutrition causes modifications to the blood tissue, hampering the development and maturation of hematopoietic cells, and these changes could be the cause of anemia, leukopenia, and bone marrow hypoplasia [1].

Protein malnutrition can disrupt numerous processes in hematopoiesis, causing damage to the hematopoietic niche, stromal cells, and the extracellular matrix, and they can result in cell death in bone marrow [1]. However, these issues are not only a consequence of inadequate nutrient supply. Here, we analyze how protein intake, in particular, caseins, the main proteinaceous component of milk, can exert numerous hematopoietic and immunomodulatory actions in addition to performing their nutritional properties [7] from the early stages of postnatal development seemingly throughout life.

2. Casein

Milk proteins can be broadly classified into three categories: caseins, whey proteins, and mucins [8], as proteins present in the milk fat globule membrane. In milk, caseins interact with calcium phosphate, forming large stable colloidal particles termed micelles. The micelles consist of casein molecules, calcium, inorganic phosphate, and citrate ions [9]. These micelles make it possible to maintain a supersaturated calcium phosphate concentration in milk, providing the newborn with sufficient calcium phosphate for the mineralization of calcified tissues [10].

Casein (from the Latin word *caseus* for cheese) comprises the major protein component of milk of most mammals [11], but relative proportions of caseins differ widely between species. In this sense, caseins comprise approximately 80% of the total protein in ruminant milk [12], but only about 55% of the total protein in horse milk [13].

Casein, which is a phosphoprotein, contains 0.7–0.9% phosphorus that is covalently bound to the protein by serine ester linkages [9], composed of many hundreds of individual amino acids, each of which may have a positive or a negative charge depending on the pH of the milk system. All amino acids that are essential to humans are present in casein in high proportions, with the possible exception of cysteine [9]. It is widely accepted that the main physiological role of casein in the milk system is to be a source of amino acids that are required for the growth of the neonate; therefore, casein is considered a highly nutritious protein. However, the dominant physiological role of the casein micelle system is to prevent pathological calcification of the mammary gland [14]. Over time, it has been revealed that casein is a protein whose physiological importance reaches levels far superior to the food field, having a wide array of biological activities including antimicrobial activities, facilitating absorption of nutrients, as well as acting as a growth factor and an immune stimulant [15].

Caseins are consist of at least three and normally four gene products and further divided into αS1-casein, αS2-casein, β-casein, and κ-casein in farm animals [11, 16] and human, and each has slightly different properties that are caused by small variations in their amino acid content. The four different types are known to occur in at least 10 genetic variants (A1–A3 and B–H) from which the A2, A1, and B forms are the most prevalent [9].

Casein is the major component of bovine milk, whereas whey is predominant in human milk. The human milk whey/casein ratio changes over the course of lactation, declining from 90/10 in colostrum (days [d] 0–5) to 65/35 in transitional milk (d6–15), then 60/40 beginning at 1 month postpartum, and continuing throughout the first year of lactation [8].

Caseins are synthesized in the mammary gland and are under multihormonal control, and in the bovine genome, they are linked within a 200-kb region on chromosome 6, in the order αS1-, β-, αS2- and κ-casein [17].

Bovine milk caseins are composed mainly of equal amounts of β-casein and αS1-casein [11] also contains κ-caseins [18], whereas human milk contains β- and κ-casein and a low concentration of α-casein. The whey/casein ratio in the formula is similar to that of mature human milk (60/40), but the formula contains all bovine milk caseins. The concentrations of total caseins and β- and κ-casein increase slightly between early and transitional milk before declining and remaining relatively stable in mature milk. In contrast, the concentration of α-casein is constant throughout lactation [19].

αS2-casein is the most calcium-sensitive member of the casein family; the sensitivity is potentially due to its high ester phosphate content, which ranges from 10 to 13 phosphate groups per peptide chain [20]. αS2-casein comprises up to 10% of the casein fraction in bovine milk; it consists of two major and several minor components that exhibit varying levels of posttranslational phosphorylation [21] as well as minor degrees of intermolecular disulfide bonding [22]. αS1-casein is only found in trace amounts in human milk (between 3 and 540 μg/mL postpartum) [23] and is thus unlikely to function as a significant amino acid source for breastfed infants [24].

β-Casein has 209 amino acids. The presence of proline or histidine at the 67th position of β-casein allows the distinction between two types of milk, A1 and A2; otherwise, there are no other differences between the two caseins. A1 β-casein is a major variant of β-casein in the milk of the common dairy cows of north European origin: Friesian, Ayrshire, British Shorthorn, and Holstein. A2 β-casein is predominantly found in the milk of Channel Island cows, Guernsey and Jersey cows, Southern French breeds, Charolais and Limousin cows [25], and Zebu original cattle of Africa. The presence of proline or histidine at the 67th position of β-casein is associated with a major effect in terms of bioactive peptide release by different gastrointestinal enzymes [26]; thus, a bioactive seven-amino-acid peptide, β-casomorphin-7 (BCM-7), can be more easily released in the small intestine by digestion of A1 β-casein with pepsin, leucine aminopeptidase, and elastase, but the alternative proline at position 67 prevents a cleavage at this site [27].

κ-Casein contains only one cysteine residue [28, 29], which implies that it is unable to form homomultimers, but it is capable of making one intermolecular disulfide bond [10]. In bovine milk, κ-casein exists as homomultimers cross-linked by random disulfide bonds [22], and it plays a key role in maintaining the stability and solubility of the micelle. Thus, the other caseins do not seem to have a role that requires well-defined structures, and κ-casein may well be more structured to fulfill its function as the interface between the calcium-sensitive caseins and milk serum [30]. In that role, κ-casein naturally resides at the surface of the casein micelle [31].

3. Casein and hematopoietic tissue

Low protein intake can affect all systems and organs, but it primarily affects tissues with a high rate of cell turnover, such as hematopoietic tissue [6]. Recently, Hastreiter et al. [32] compared a low-protein diet based on 20 g/kg casein with a control diet based on 120 g/kg casein, and they showed that male C57BL/6 mice after the period of malnutrition presented with peripheral leukopenia and a reduction in lymphocytes and monocytes, especially in granulocytic cells associated with bone marrow hypoplasia. Therefore, hematopoietic stem cell (Lin-Sca-1+c-Kit+-LSK) and progenitor cell (CD45+CD34+) populations were decreased in malnourished animals [33], but also low protein intake induced a specific reduction in granulocyte-monocyte progenitors (Lin-IL7r-c-Kit+Sca-1-CD16/32^{high}), which explains, in part, why there was a reduction in mature granulocytes [32].

It is well known that in protein malnutrition states, the number of granulocytic cells, especially neutrophils, is reduced, which predisposes patients to higher susceptibility to infection [34, 35]. However, this involvement in hematopoiesis cannot be explained only because there are not enough amino acids to support the requirements of an expanding tissue; other cellular mechanisms are involved. In this sense, Hastreiter et al. showed that there is an impaired ability of c-Kit+ cells from the bone marrow of malnourished animals to produce CFU-GEMM and CFU-GM cells, which are myeloid progenitors and, consequently, are the cells responsible for granulopoiesis [36]; this malfunction is related to Kit+ cells exhibiting reduced expression of the receptor of granulocyte colony-stimulating factor (G-CSFr), which is a granulopoietic cytokine [32].

Interestingly, Domínguez-Melendez et al. showed that administration of casein as sodium caseinate in BALB/c mice increased the percentage of myeloid precursors from bone marrow and increased the total number of bone marrow leukocytes resulting from cell proliferation. They also found that casein induced proliferation and activation of granulocytes, and it increased the serum concentration of cytokines such as G-CSF, M-CSF, and GM-CSF [37]. These cytokines are key to the proliferation, differentiation, and activation of granulomonocytic cells, which in turn induce multiple functions within the immune response; since these cytokines regulate inflammation, as is the case for monocyte-macrophages, they are responsible for phagocytosis, which is a crucial event in fungal and bacterial infections; once activated, macrophages are the bridge between activated CD4+ lymphocytes and the adaptive immune response [38]. For the lymphoid lineage in vivo, sodium caseinate also influences the induction of IL-7, a key cytokine involved in lymphopoiesis of B cells, which are key cells for the adaptive immune response, since once activated, they are responsible for producing antibodies that they will opsonize foreign antigens to facilitate their elimination [39].

This suggests that casein may be linked to the development of the immune system in the early stages of life, and it may be relevant throughout life as a way of activating the immune system; this notion has been demonstrated experimentally by mice that, when injected with lethal doses of bacteria, can survive only after inducing protection by granulocytes with administration of casein [40].

Studies of the effect of casein or sodium caseinate on hematopoietic tissue in vivo and in vitro are limited, and most of them do not include non-casein protein experimental controls. In some cases, there could be controversy in its effects observed due to the presence of a general source of protein or if they were specific to casein. In this sense, it would be more than advisable for future casein work to consider the inclusion of non-casein protein controls.

4. The role of caseins in granulopoiesis and monocytopoiesis

Caseins and sodium caseinate have been studied for almost four decades, where, from the beginning, it was clear that there was a proinflammatory effect of casein on myeloid lineage cells; this activity was demonstrated by Lotem and Sachs working group, which showed that sodium caseinate had the ability to differentiate a leukemic cell line of myeloid origin toward granulocytes and macrophages in mice via inflammation and via the activity of T lymphocytes in the peritoneal cavity [41]. Later, this same group showed that the inflammation caused by sodium caseinate had the ability to induce the production of G-CSF and GM-CSF in vitro and in vivo [42]. Another study showed that protein deprivation, such as dietary casein restriction, in rats directly resulted in a decrease in erythropoietin, which is a hormone that is directly related to the proliferation of the erythroid lineage [43]. In a similar study, the role of casein on this lineage was reconfirmed, since the restriction of protein in standard diets in mice once again demonstrated the involvement of proteins in the proliferation of erythroid progenitors in mice [44]. Subsequently, it was shown that after intraperitoneal inoculation of casein, both the production of G-CSF and GM-CSF were rapidly induced, and the high concentration of both cytokines caused a high migration of neutrophils only at the site of inoculation, but they revealed no increase in their percentage in the bone marrow [45]. Interestingly, in a study carried out by the Noursadeghi group, it was shown that after previous inoculation of casein, protection could be given to mice treated with lethal doses of bacteria, and this was due to defensive ability of activated neutrophils recruited by G-CSF induced by that intraperitoneal (IP) injection of casein [40]. Regarding the casein and sodium caseinate fractions on myeloid cell lines, one study showed that in vitro sodium caseinate had the ability to inhibit the proliferation of a myeloid cell line 32D without inhibiting its viability. On the other hand, α-casein exhibited the ability to inhibit the proliferation of a myeloid tumor line, which is the case for WEHI-3 and sodium caseinate of tumor lines J-774 and P388 at different concentrations. In this same study, it was shown that casein fractions α-, β- and κ-casein could induce differentiation of the 32D cell line but not the WEHI-3 tumor cell line, but the study interestingly demonstrated that sodium caseinate and a-casein have the ability to induce M-CSF secretion in the 32D cell line [46]. The same group of researchers subsequently demonstrated that sodium caseinate has the ability to induce the differentiation of the granulocytic lineage in vitro in the same way that G-CSF does, and G-CSF is the specific cytokine required for the differentiation of this lineage; these results demonstrated that these cells have the ability to induce the production of functional M-CSF, a key cytokine in the activation and differentiation of the monocytic lineage [47]. The Vordenbaumen group demonstrated that macrophages of human origin could be stimulated by human αS1-casein to produce GM-CSF and that αS1-casein activated the p38 MAPK pathway, which is an important signal in cells of hematopoietic origin. Interestingly, this group found that αS1-casein was linked to specific receptors for the protein in most of the macrophages analyzed and not only that but also that it could induce the production of IL-1 and IL-6, which positions it as an excellent immunomodulatory protein [48]. This same group subsequently demonstrated that αS1-casein in human milk has the ability to differentiate human monocytes from macrophages, and they also increase the phagocytic capacity of the monocytes in vitro once stimulated with the protein [49]. On the other hand, the Santiago-Osorio group showed that the IP inoculation of BALB/c mice with sodium caseinate induces in vivo proliferation of the myeloid lineage in the bone marrow. Interestingly, it was observed that the granulocytes had the ability to incorporate BrdU, a thymidine analyte that is incorporated into proliferating cells; further, the cells exhibited a greater ability to phagocytose when compared to cells from mice that had not received treatment [37].

5. The role of caseins in lymphopoiesis

Regarding the influence of caseins or sodium caseinate on the lymphoid lineage, the role of these proteins is not prominent, but they have interesting functions in vivo and in vitro; for instance, the proteolytic activity of leukocytes can be induced by β-casein in vitro [50]. In another work, it was demonstrated that peptides derived from αS1-casein increased the concentration of IFN-γ by stimulating CD8+ T cells, and IFN-γ is a potent inhibitor of Th2 lymphocyte-dependent events as well as an inhibitor of the production of IgE [51]. Another working group demonstrated that β-casein rather than κ-casein is mainly responsible for inhibiting spleen CD3+ T lymphocytes [52]. In a more detailed work, the group of Santiago Osorio demonstrated that the IP inoculation of BALB/c mice with sodium caseinate decreases the proliferation of B/B220+ lymphocytes in bone marrow, but this lineage increases proliferation in the spleen; this observation suggests that the IP injection induces extramedullary lymphopoiesis, while the treatment does not increase the proliferation of lineage lymphocytes specifically in the thymus and has only very subtle effects in the spleen without affecting the viability of both lineages. It should be noted that the production of IL-2, IL-7, and IL-15 is increased, and they are key interleukins involved in lymphopoiesis of both T cells and B cells in mice [53]. Although there is currently clear evidence for the role of caseins or sodium caseinate on the lymphoid lineage, there is more evidence of their effect on the myeloid lineage, which may be due to the characteristics of the protein and its particular influence on these cells. However, the field is still open to further exploration of the role of sodium caseinate or caseins on the lymphoid lineage, since its role is not yet clear.

6. Inflammation and immune system enhancement by caseins

Milk is a complex physiological liquid that simultaneously provides nutrients and bioactive components, including prebiotics, immune proteins, and the microbiome of human milk itself; the establishment of symbiotic microflora and the development of gut-associated lymphoid tissues facilitate the successful postnatal adaptation of the newborn infant by stimulating cellular growth and digestive maturation [9]. Breastfeeding is associated with a decreased incidence of gastrointestinal (GI) tract infections [54, 55], which is corroborated by several studies that have correlated breastfeeding with a lower incidence of necrotizing enterocolitis in humans and animal models [56, 57].

The antimicrobial activity in milk is greater than the sum individual immunoglobulin and of whey proteins such as lactoferrin, lactoferricins, lactoperoxidase, lysozyme, lactenin, casecudubs, etc. [58]; this activity could be also associated with gut-colonizing bacteria that prevent adhesion and colonization of pathogenic bacteria while stimulating mucosal cell proliferation and enhancing immune development [59]; a portion of these antimicrobial activities are performed by caseins, most likely κ-casein fucose carbohydrate residues.

Purified human κ-casein inhibits specific adhesion of *Helicobacter pylori* to mucous cells at the human gastric surface. The inhibitory activity is abolished by the oxidation of metaperiodate and is considerably reduced by preincubation with alpha-L-fucosidase but not with α-N-acetylneuraminidase or endo-β-galactosidase. Thus, glycosylated κ-casein is likely important for the inhibition of *Helicobacter pylori* adhesion and, therefore, infection. This could explain why breastfeeding may protect against *Helicobacter pylori* infection during early life and how the species-specific glycosylation patterns in human bovine κ-casein partly determine both the narrow host spectrum of this human gastric pathogen and the capacity to resist infection [60].

Unphosphorylated αS1-casein in breast milk may contribute to the development of the immune system before major colonization of the gut by microbes occurs by triggering immune responses to potential pathogens, including pathogen-associated molecules such as LPS. Moreover, αS1-casein by itself gives rise to sustained specific IgG antibody production in individuals who nursed [61]. Early infantile autoantibody production in turn is speculated to confer protection from pathogens [62].

αS1-casein activates the secretion of the proinflammatory cytokines GM-CSF (granulocyte-macrophage colony-stimulating factor), IL1-β (interleukin 1β), IL-6 (interleukin 6), and chemokine IL-8 (interleukin 8) in human monocytes via the mitogen-activated protein kinase p38 (MAPK-p38) signaling pathway [24, 49].

Human unphosphorylated αS1-casein induces Toll-like receptor 4 (TLRs) mediated expression of the proinflammatory cytokines IL-1β, GM-CSF, and IL-6 in monocytic cells [63] and induces the differentiation of monocytes toward macrophages [49, 64], but this process is not dependent upon LPS. Interestingly, a posttranslational modification in αS1-casein (a phosphorylation event) inhibits binding to TLR4, which acts as an off switch for proinflammatory effects [48]. Ectopic expression (outside the mammary gland) of αS1-casein has been detected in inflamed tissues such as synovial cells and cartilage of rheumatoid arthritis, osteoarthritis, and multiple sclerosis patients [63, 65–67], prostate hyperplasia [68], and lymph nodes of encephalomyelitic mice [67]. Hence, αS1-casein may constitute an autogenous stimulus that upholds chronic autoimmune inflammation via TLR4 [64].

On the other hand, it is known that casein and sodium caseinate are agents that can induce inflammation when inoculated intraperitoneally, and it has been shown that sodium caseinate and casein can stimulate neutrophils to produce proinflammatory cytokines, such as M-CSF, in vitro [47]. Not only that, but it is known that they can induce in this same lineage signaling pathways involved in inflammation, such as p38 MAPK, which in turn stimulates the production of key cytokines both in inflammation and in hematopoietic cell differentiation processes [69]. However, casein inoculation can induce a rapid accumulation of neutrophils within 3 h due to selective release of mature cells from the bone marrow; then, a significant increase in the concentrations of granulocyte-macrophage colony-stimulating factor (GM-CSF) and granulocyte colony-stimulating factor (G-CSF) occurs in the peritoneal cavity [45], but the accumulation did not affect the serum values of TNF-α, IL-1β, or IL-6. As demonstrated by Noursadeghi, inflammation induced by casein was associated with higher serum G-CSF concentrations, and administration of an Ab that neutralized this cytokine completely nullified protection against *Escherichia coli* infection after casein pretreatment. Injection of recombinant murine G-CSF between 3 and 24 h before infection conferred the same protection that was provided by casein injection [40].

7. Toll-like receptors (TLRs) and caseins

Caseins serve as a source of amino acids but also perform a range of functions, including improving micronutrient bioavailability, stimulating intestinal growth and maturation, supporting immunologic defense, shaping the microbiome, and enhancing learning and memory [19]. Some bioactive peptides in milk act in variable ways as antihypertensives, antithrombotic agents, opioids, antimicrobials, cytomodulators, and immunomodulators [70]. How can this be possible, if proteins are degraded in the gastrointestinal tract to yield the essential amino acids for the development of the neonate?

Bioactive milk peptides were first described in 1950, when Mellander (1950) reported that ingestion of casein-derived phosphorylated peptides led to enhanced vitamin D-independent calcification in rachitic infants. While bioactive peptides can be generated from a variety of foods, milk proteins are generally regarded as a very rich source; as a result, they have become fundamental constituents of several commercially available functional food products and ingredients [19].

What is the bridge that connects casein, the genesis of myeloid and lymphoid hematopoietic cells, and the activation of the immune system? This linking role may be the direct responsibility of TLRs, which are receptors that recognize at least α-casein and β-casein [71] and are expressed in granulocytes, macrophages, and B and T lymphocytes; TLRs are capable of activating these cells to produce key cytokines for both proliferation and activation of the innate and adaptive immune response, such as TNF-α [72], G-CSF, IL-2 [73, 74], and IL-7 [75].

In this sense, there is evidence that at least β-casein can influence B lymphocytes via TLR4 [76, 77], and a recent study showed that casein binds directly to TLR4 of CD8+ T lymphocytes [64], although it has also been shown that β-casein can influence the activation and production of histamine through a kinase-dependent mechanism PI3 [78].

Regarding the role of TLR in the production of key cytokines for the activation and proliferation of both T and B lymphocytes, TLR4 of T lymphocytes is involved in the production of IL-2 [73, 74].

For myeloid cells, neutrophils have been shown to use both TLR4 and TLR2 for survival and activation [79]. Thus, TRL4 is essential for the production of G-CSF in neutrophils stimulated with *Clostridium* [80], and another study showed that in addition to G-CSF, TLR4 is capable of inducing the expression of GM-CSF, which plays a fundamental role in the activation and differentiation of both neutrophils and monocytes [81].

TLRs have been shown to be essential for the activation of monocytic cells, and it plays a role in the production of GM-CSF by activating the transcription factor PU.I, which plays a fundamental role in this lineage [82]. In dendritic cells derived from macrophages, TLRs are involved in the synthesis of IL-7, which is an essential interleukin for the maintenance of LT CD8+ [75]. Therefore, casein or sodium

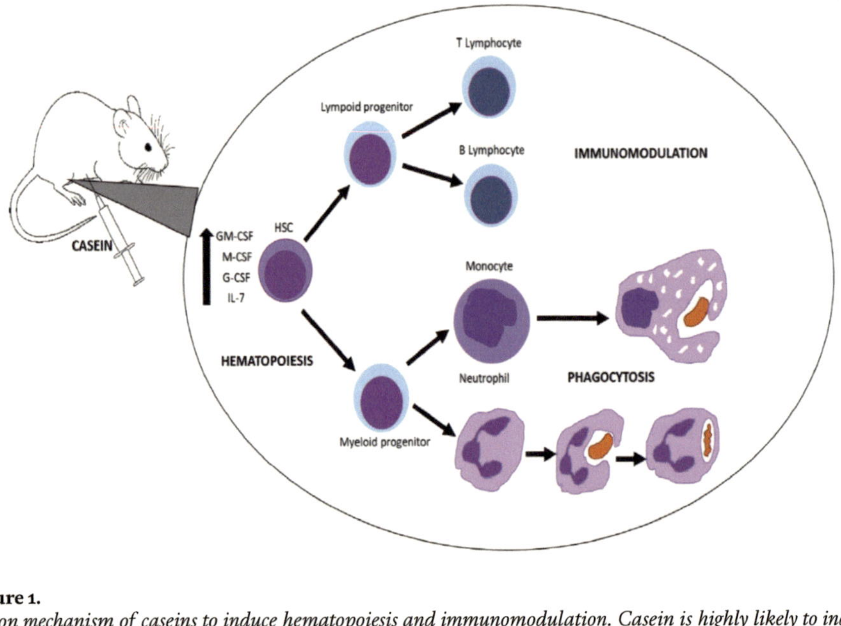

Figure 1.
Action mechanism of caseins to induce hematopoiesis and immunomodulation. Casein is highly likely to induce TLR4 activation, after which the expression of GM-CSF, G-CSF, M-CSF, and IL-7 is induced in both myeloid and lymphoid cells. This massive cellular activation of hematopoietic cells and immune responses explain the antimicrobial and immunomodulatory effects of casein.

caseinate could stimulate TLR4 via the production of at least IL-7 in dendritic cells derived from macrophages.

It is clear that there is a close relationship between TLR4 and cells of myeloid and lymphoid origin, as these cells use TLR4 both in their proliferation and in their activation. This relationship then entails the production of cytokines of myeloid and lymphoid origin, and these cytokines in turn are key pieces for the proliferation and activation of these same cells. Thus, TLR4-bound caseins or sodium caseinate are highly likely to induce TLR4 activation, after which the expression of GM-CSF, G-CSF, M-CSF, and IL-7 is induced in both myeloid and lymphoid cells (**Figure 1**). It is even possible that indirectly, by stimulating other cell types, TLR4 could induce the activation of cells that can influence the erythroid and megakaryocyte lineage. Then, this massive cellular activation of hematopoietic cells and immune responses could explain the antimicrobial and immunomodulatory effects of casein as well as the activity of casein as an antihypertensive, antithrombotic, and antioxidant molecule [83].

Here, we can reveal that activation of the innate immune system by casein could be useful to fight pathogens resistant to antibiotics, as has been suggested [40], so casein could be used to induce a strong immune response in immunosuppressed patients [84, 85]; it could be used as a prophylactic strategy to prevent infections.

Acknowledgements

This work was financially supported by DGAPA PAPIIT IN221017 & IN229820.

Author details

Edgar Ledesma-Martinez[1], Vanihamin Domínguez-Meléndez[2], Itzen Aguiñiga-Sánchez[1] and Edelmiro Santiago-Osorio[1*]

1 Hematopoiesis and Leukemia Laboratory, Research Unit on Cell Differentiation and Cancer, FES Zaragoza, National Autonomous University of Mexico, Mexico City, Mexico

2 Center for Health Studies and Services (CESS), University of Veracruz, Veracruz City, Mexico

*Address all correspondence to: edelmiro@unam.mx

References

[1] Santos EW, Oliveira DC, Silva GB, Tsujita M, Beltran JO, Hastreiter A, et al. Hematological alterations in protein malnutrition. Nutrition Reviews. 2017;**75**:909-919. DOI: 10.1093/nutrit/nux041

[2] Wilkinson AC, Yamazaki S. The hematopoietic stem cell diet. International Journal of Hematology. 2018;**107**:634-641. DOI: 10.1007/s12185-018-2451-1

[3] Mana MD, Kuo EYS, Yilmaz ÖH. Dietary regulation of adult stem cells. Current Stem Cell Reports. 2017;**3**:1-8. DOI: 10.1007/s40778-017-0072-x

[4] Lazare S, Ausema A, Reijne AC, van Dijk G, van Os R, de Haan G. Lifelong dietary intervention does not affect hematopoietic stem cell function. Experimental Hematology. 2017;**53**:26-30. DOI: 10.1016/j.exphem.2017.06.002

[5] Mihaylova MM, Sabatini DM, Yilmaz ÖH. Dietary and metabolic control of stem cell function in physiology and cancer. Cell Stem Cell. 2014;**14**:292-305. DOI: 10.1016/j.stem.2014.02.008

[6] Borelli P, Blatt SL, Rogero MM, Fock RA. Haematological alterations in protein malnutrition. Revista Brasileira de Hematologia e Hemoterapia. 2004;**26**:49-56. DOI: 10.1590/s1516-84842004000100010

[7] Hvatum M, Kanerud L, Hällgren R, Brandtzaeg P. The gut-joint axis: Cross reactive food antibodies in rheumatoid arthritis. Gut. 2006;**55**:1240-1247. DOI: 10.1136/gut.2005.076901

[8] Lönnerdal B, Erdmann P, Thakkar SK, Sauser J, Destaillats F. Longitudinal evolution of true protein, amino acids and bioactive proteins in breast milk: A developmental perspective. The Journal of Nutritional Biochemistry. 2017;**41**:1-11. DOI: 10.1016/j.jnutbio.2016.06.001

[9] Petrotos K, Tsakali E, Goulas P, D'Alessandro AG. Casein and whey proteins in human health. In: Milk and Dairy Products as Functional Foods. 2014:94-146. DOI: 10.1002/9781118635056.ch4

[10] Johnsen LB, Rasmussen LK, Petersen TE, Berglund L. Characterization of three types of human α(s1)-casein mRNA transcripts. Biochemical Journal. 1995;**309**:237-242. DOI: 10.1042/bj3090237

[11] Ginger MR, Grigor MR. Comparative aspects of milk caseins. Comparative Biochemistry and Physiology. Part B, Biochemistry & Molecular Biology. 1999;**124**:133-145. DOI: 10.1016/s0305-0491(99)00110-8

[12] Wang X, Zhao X, Huang D, Pan X, Qi Y, Yang Y, et al. Proteomic analysis and cross species comparison of casein fractions from the milk of dairy animals. Scientific Reports. 2017;**7**:1-9. DOI: 10.1038/srep43020

[13] Uniacke-Lowe T, Fox PF. Equine milk proteins: Chemistry, structure and nutritional significance. International Dairy Journal. 2010;**20**:609-629. DOI: 10.1016/J.IDAIRYJ.2010.02.007

[14] Holt C. The milk salts and their interaction with casein. In: Adv. Dairy Chem. Vol. 3. Springer US; 1997. pp. 233-256. DOI: 10.1007/978-1-4757-4409-5_6

[15] Mølgaard C, Larnkjær A, Arnberg K, Michaelsen KF. Milk and growth in children: Effects of whey and casein. In: Nestle Nutr. Work. Ser. Pediatr. Progr. Basel: KARGER; 2011. pp. 67-78. DOI: 10.1159/000325576

[16] Holt C, Carver JA, Ecroyd H, Thorn DC. Invited review: Caseins and the

casein micelle: Their biological functions, structures, and behavior in foods 1. Journal of Dairy Science. 2013;**96**:6127-6146. DOI: 10.3168/jds.2013-6831

[17] Ferretti L, Leone P, Sgaramella V. Long range restriction analysis of the bovine casein genes. Nucleic Acids Research. 1990;**18**:6829-6833. DOI: 10.1093/nar/18.23.6829

[18] Day L, Williams RPW, Otter D, Augustin MA. Casein polymorphism heterogeneity influences casein micelle size in milk of individual cows. Journal of Dairy Science. 2015;**98**:3633-3644. DOI: 10.3168/jds.2014-9285

[19] Donovan SM. Human Milk Proteins: Composition and Physiological Significance. 2019. pp. 93-101. DOI: 10.1159/000490298

[20] Farrell HM, Jimenez-Flores R, Bleck GT, Brown EM, Butler JE, Creamer LK, et al. Nomenclature of the proteins of cows' milk—Sixth revision. Journal of Dairy Science. 2004;**87**:1641-1674. DOI: 10.3168/jds.S0022-0302(04)73319-6

[21] Swaisgood HE. Chemistry of the caseins. In: Advanced Dairy Chemistry—1 Proteins. Boston, MA: Springer; 1992. pp. 63-110

[22] Rasmussen LK, Hojrup P, Petersen TE. Localization of two interchain disulfide bridges in dimers of bovine alpha s2-casein. Parallel and antiparallel alignments of the polypeptide chains. European Journal of Biochemistry. 1992;**203**:381-386. DOI: 10.1111/j.1432-1033.1992.tb16561.x

[23] Altendorfer I, König S, Braukmann A, Saenger T, Bleck E, Vordenbäumen S, et al. Quantification of αS1-casein in breast milk using a targeted mass spectrometry-based approach. Journal of Pharmaceutical and Biomedical Analysis. 2015;**103**:52-58. DOI: 10.1016/j.jpba.2014.10.034

[24] Vordenbäumen S, Braukmann A, Petermann K, Scharf A, Bleck E, von Mikecz A, et al. Casein αs1 is expressed by human monocytes and upregulates the production of GM-CSF via p 38 MAPK. Journal of Immunology. 2011;**186**:592-601. DOI: 10.4049/jimmunol.1001461

[25] Ng-Kwai-Hang K, Grosclaude F. Genetic polymorphism of milk proteins. In: Advanced Dairy Chemistry. Boston, MA: Springer; 1992

[26] Ul Haq MR, Kapila R, Shandilya UK, Kapila S. Impact of milk derived β-casomorphins on physiological functions and trends in research: A review. International Journal of Food Properties. 2014;**17**:1726-1741. DOI: 10.1080/10942912.2012.712077

[27] Truswell AS. The A2 milk case: A critical review. European Journal of Clinical Nutrition. 2005;**59**:623-631. DOI: 10.1038/sj.ejcn.1602104

[28] Brignon G, Chtourou A, Ribadeau-Dumas B. Preparation and amino acid sequence of human κ-casein. FEBS Letters. 1985;**188**:48-54. DOI: 10.1016/0014-5793(85)80872-3

[29] Bergström S, Hansson L, Hernell O, Lönnerdal B, Nilsson AK, Strömqvist M. Cloning and sequencing of human k-casein cDNA. Mitochondrial DNA. 1992;**3**:245-246. DOI: 10.3109/10425179209034024

[30] Creamer LK, Plowman JE, Liddell MJ, Smith MH, Hill JP. Micelle stability: κ-casein structure and function. Journal of Dairy Science. 1998;**81**:3004-3012. DOI: 10.3168/jds.S0022-0302(98)75864-3

[31] Holt C. Structure and stability of bovine casein micelles. Advances in Protein Chemistry. 1992;**43**:63-151. DOI: 10.1016/S0065-3233(08)60554-9

[32] Hastreiter AA, Makiyama EN, Borelli P, Fock RA. Impairment of

G-CSF receptor on granulocytic progenitor cells causes neutropenia in protein malnutrition. Nutrition. 2020;**69**:1-8. DOI: 10.1016/j.nut.2019.06.021

[33] Livak KJ, Schmittgen TD. Analysis of relative gene expression data using real-time quantitative PCR and the 2-ΔΔCT method. Methods. 2001;**25**:402-408. DOI: 10.1006/meth.2001.1262

[34] Scrimshaw NS, Viteri FE. INCAP studies of kwashiorkor and marasmus. Food and Nutrition Bulletin. 2010;**31**:34-41. DOI: 10.1177/156482651003100105

[35] Keusch GT. The history of nutrition: Malnutrition, infection and immunity. The Journal of Nutrition. 2003;**133**:336S-340S. DOI: 10.1093/jn/133.1.336s

[36] Chee LCY, Hendy J, Purton LE, McArthur GA. The granulocyte-colony stimulating factor receptor (G-CSFR) interacts with retinoic acid receptors (RARs) in the regulation of myeloid differentiation. Journal of Leukocyte Biology. 2013;**93**:235-243. DOI: 10.1189/jlb.1211609

[37] Domínguez-Melendez V, Silvestre-Santana O, Moreno-Fierros L, Aguiñiga-Sánchez I, Martínez L, Marroquin-Segura R, et al. Sodium caseinate induces mouse granulopoiesis. Inflammation Research. 2012;**61**:367-373. DOI: 10.1007/s00011-011-0421-7

[38] Harmon JR, Spengler JR, Coleman-McCray JD, Nichol ST, Spiropoulou CF, McElroy AK. CD4 T cells, CD8 T cells, and monocytes coordinate to prevent rift valley fever virus encephalitis. Journal of Virology. 2018;**92**:e01270-18. DOI: 10.1128/jvi.01270-18

[39] Sawa T, Kinoshita M, Inoue K, Ohara J, Moriyama K. Immunoglobulin for treating bacterial infections: One more mechanism of action. Antibodies. 2019;**8**:52. DOI: 10.3390/antib8040052

[40] Noursadeghi M, Bickerstaff MCM, Herbert J, Moyes D, Cohen J, Pepys MB. Production of granulocyte colony-stimulating factor in the nonspecific acute phase response enhances host resistance to bacterial infection. Journal of Immunology. 2002;**169**:913-919. DOI: 10.4049/jimmunol.169.2.913

[41] Lotem J, Sachs L. Control of in vivo differentiation of myeloid leukemic cells. III. Regulation by T lymphocytes and inflammation. International Journal of Cancer. 1983;**32**:781-791. DOI: 10.1002/ijc.2910320620

[42] Lotem J, Sachs L. Independent regulation of myeloid cell growth and differentiation inducing proteins: In vivo regulation by compounds that induce inflammation. International Journal of Cancer. 1985;**35**:93-100. DOI: 10.1002/ijc.2910350115

[43] Okano M, Ohnota H, Sasaki R. Protein deficiency impairs erythropoiesis in rats by reducing serum erythropoietin concentration and the population size of erythroid precursor cells. The Journal of Nutrition. 1992;**122**:1376-1383. DOI: 10.1093/jn/122.7.1376

[44] Barceló AC, Alippi RM, Boyer P, Olivera MI, Mide SM, Caro J, et al. Impaired response of polycythemic mice to erythropoietin induced by protein starvation imposed after hormone administration. Stem Cells. 1993;**11**:296-302. DOI: 10.1002/stem.5530110407

[45] Metcalf D, Robb L, Dunn AR, Mifsud S, Di Rago L. Role of granulocyte-macrophage colony-stimulating factor and granulocyte colony-stimulating factor in the development of an acute neutrophil inflammatory response in mice. Blood.

1996;**88**:3755-3764. DOI: 10.1182/blood.v88.10.3755.bloodjournal88103755

[46] Ramos-Mandujano G, Weiss-Steider B, Melo B, Córdova Y, Ledesma-Martínez E, Bustos S, et al. Alpha-, beta- and kappa-caseins inhibit the proliferation of the myeloid cell lines 32D cl3 and WEHI-3 and exhibit different differentiation properties. Immunobiology. 2008;**213**:133-141. DOI: 10.1016/j.imbio.2007.07.004

[47] Santiago-Osorio E, Mora L, Bautista M, Montesinos JJ, Martínez I, Ramos-Mandujano G, et al. Sodium caseinate induces secretion of macrophage colony-stimulating factor from neutrophils. Immunobiology. 2010;**215**:332-339. DOI: 10.1016/j.imbio.2009.03.003

[48] Vordenbäumen S, Saenger T, Braukmann A, Tahan T, Bleck E, Jose J, et al. Human casein alpha s1 induces proinflammatory cytokine expression in monocytic cells by TLR4 signaling. Molecular Nutrition & Food Research. 2016;**60**:1079-1089. DOI: 10.1002/mnfr.201500792

[49] Vordenbäumen S, Braukmann A, Altendorfer I, Bleck E, Jose J, Schneider M. Human casein alpha s1 (CSN1S1) skews in vitro differentiation of monocytes towards macrophages. BMC Immunology. 2013;**14**:46. DOI: 10.1186/1471-2172-14-46

[50] Verdi RJ, Barbano DM. Properties of proteases from milk somatic cells and blood leukocytes. Journal of Dairy Science. 1991;**74**:2077-2081. DOI: 10.3168/jds.S0022-0302(91)78379-3

[51] Totsuka M, Kakehi M, Kohyama M, Hachimura S, Hisatsune T, Kaminogawa S.Enhancement of antigen-specific IFN-γ production from CD8+ T cells by a single amino acid-substituted peptide derived from bovine α(s1)-casein. Clinical Immunology and Immunopathology. 1998;**88**:277-286. DOI: 10.1006/clin.1998.4585

[52] Bonomi F, Brandt R, Favalli S, Ferranti P, Fierro O, Frøkiær H, et al. Structural determinants of the immunomodulatory properties of the C-terminal region of bovine β-casein. International Dairy Journal. 2011;**21**:770-776. DOI: 10.1016/j.idairyj.2011.04.012

[53] Domínguez-Meléndez V, Aguiñiga-Sánchez I, Moreno-Fierros L, Torres B, Osorio ES. El caseinato de sodio incrementa número de linfocitos B en ratones. Biomédica. 2017;**37**:571-576. DOI: 10.7705/biomedica.v34i2.3604

[54] Gill HS, Doull F, Rutherfurd KJ, Cross ML. Immunoregulatory peptides in bovine milk. British Journal of Nutrition. 2018;**84**:111-117. DOI: 10.1017/S0007114500002336

[55] M. Knopfler, How Compatible is Cow' s Milk with the Human Immune System?, 2016. Available from: https://touroscholar.touro.edu/sjlcas [Accessed: 31 January 2020]

[56] Meinzen-Derr J, Poindexter B, Wrage L, Morrow AL, Stoll B, Donovan EF. Role of human milk in extremely low birth weight infants' risk of necrotizing enterocolitis or death. Journal of Perinatology. 2009;**29**:57-62. DOI: 10.1038/jp.2008.117

[57] Sodhi C, Richardson W, Gribar S, Hackam DJ. The development of animal models for the study of necrotizing enterocolitis. Disease Models & Mechanisms. 2008;**1**:94-98. DOI: 10.1242/dmm.000315

[58] Park YW. Bioactive peptides in milk and dairy products: A review. Korean Journal for Food Science of Animal Resources. 2015;**35**:831-840. DOI: 10.5851/kosfa.2015.35.6.831

[59] Ward TL, Hosid S, Ioshikhes I, Altosaar I. Human milk metagenome: A functional capacity analysis.

BMC Microbiology. 2013;**13**:1. DOI: 10.1186/1471-2180-13-116

[60] Hernell O, Hansson L. Human milk k-casein and inhibition of helicobacter pylori adhesion to human gastric mucosa. Journal of Pediatric Gastroenterology and Nutrition. 1995;**21**:288-296. DOI: 10.1097/00005176-199510000-00006

[61] Petermann K, Vordenbäumen S, Maas R, Braukmann A, Bleck E, Saenger T, et al. Autoantibodies to αs1-casein are induced by breast-feeding. PLoS One. 2012;**7**:e32716. DOI: 10.1371/journal.pone.0032716

[62] Barbouche R, Forveille M, Fischer A, Avrameas S, Durandy A. Spontaneous IgM autoantibody production in vitro by B lymphocytes of normal human neonates. Scandinavian Journal of Immunology. 1992;**35**:659-667. DOI: 10.1111/j.1365-3083.1992.tb02972.x

[63] Galligan CL, Baig E, Bykerk V, Keystone EC, Fish EN. Distinctive gene expression signatures in rheumatoid arthritis synovial tissue fibroblast cells: Correlates with disease activity. Genes and Immunity. 2007;**8**:480-491. DOI: 10.1038/sj.gene.6364400

[64] Saenger T, Vordenbäumen S, Genich S, Haidar S, Schulte M, Nienberg C, et al. Human αS1-casein induces IL-8 secretion by binding to the ecto-domain of the TLR4/MD2 receptor complex. Biochimica et Biophysica Acta, General Subjects. 2019;**1863**:632-643. DOI: 10.1016/j.bbagen.2018.12.007

[65] Ungethuem U, Haeupl T, Witt H, Koczan D, Krenn V, Huber H, et al. Molecular signatures and new candidates to target the pathogenesis of rheumatoid arthritis. Physiological Genomics. 2010;**42A**:267-282. DOI: 10.1152/physiolgenomics.00004.2010

[66] Karlsson C, Dehne T, Lindahl A, Brittberg M, Pruss A, Sittinger M, et al. Genome-wide expression profiling reveals new candidate genes associated with osteoarthritis. Osteoarthritis and Cartilage. 2010;**18**:581-592. DOI: 10.1016/j.joca.2009.12.002

[67] Otaegui D, Mostafavi S, Bernard CCA, de Munain AL, Mousavi P, Oksenberg JR, et al. Increased transcriptional activity of milk-related genes following the active phase of experimental autoimmune encephalomyelitis and multiple sclerosis. Journal of Immunology. 2007;**179**:4074-4082. DOI: 10.4049/jimmunol.179.6.4074

[68] Xu K, Ling MT, Wang X, Wong YC. Evidence of a novel biomarker, αs1-Casein, a milk protein, in benign prostate hyperplasia. Prostate Cancer and Prostatic Diseases. 2006;**9**:293-297. DOI: 10.1038/sj.pcan.4500872

[69] Van Overmeire E, Stijlemans B, Heymann F, Keirsse J, Morias Y, Elkrim Y, et al. M-CSF and GM-CSF receptor signaling differentially regulate monocyte maturation and macrophage polarization in the tumor microenvironment. Cancer Research. 2016;**76**:35-42. DOI: 10.1158/0008-5472.CAN-15-0869

[70] Hayes M, Stanton C, Fitzgerald GF, Ross RP. Putting microbes to work: Dairy fermentation, cell factories and bioactive peptides. Part II: Bioactive peptide functions. Biotechnology Journal. 2007;**2**:435-449. DOI: 10.1002/biot.200700045

[71] Lewis SL, Van Epps DE. Demonstration of specific receptors for fluoresceinated casein on human neutrophils and monocytes using flow cytometry. Inflammation. 1983;**7**:363-375. DOI: 10.1007/BF00916301

[72] Arruda-Silva F, Bianchetto-Aguilera F, Gasperini S, Polletti S, Cosentino E, Tamassia N, et al. Human neutrophils produce CCL23 in response to various TLR-agonists and TNFα. Frontiers in Cellular and Infection

Microbiology. 2017;7:176. DOI: 10.3389/fcimb.2017.00176

[73] Rossato L, dos Santos SS, Ferreira LG, de Almeida SR. The importance of Toll-like receptor 4 during experimental *Sporothrix brasiliensis* infection. Medical Mycology. 2019;**57**:489-495. DOI: 10.1093/mmy/myy048

[74] Seydoux E, Liang H, Dubois Cauwelaert N, Archer M, Rintala ND, Kramer R, et al. Effective combination adjuvants engage both TLR and inflammasome pathways to promote potent adaptive immune responses. Journal of Immunology. 2018;**201**:98-112. DOI: 10.4049/jimmunol.1701604

[75] Carreno BM, Becker-Hapak M, Linette GP. CD40 regulates human dendritic cell-derived IL-7 production that, in turn, contributes to $CD8^+$ T-cell antigen-specific expansion. Immunology and Cell Biology. 2009;**87**:167-177. DOI: 10.1038/icb.2008.80

[76] Tobita K, Kawahara T, Otani H. Bovine β-casein (1-28), a casein phosphopeptide, enhances proliferation and IL-6 expression of mouse CD19+ cells via toll-like receptor 4. Journal of Agricultural and Food Chemistry. 2006;**54**:8013-8017. DOI: 10.1021/jf0610864

[77] Kawahara T, Katayama D, Otani H. Effect of-casein (1-28) on proliferative responses and secretory functions of human immunocompetent cell lines. Bioscience, Biotechnology, and Biochemistry. 2004;**68**:2091-2095

[78] Smuda C, Wechsler JB, Bryce PJ. TLR-induced activation of neutrophils promotes histamine production via a PI3 kinase dependent mechanism. Immunology Letters. 2011;**141**:102-108. DOI: 10.1016/j.imlet.2011.08.002

[79] Sabroe I, Prince LR, Jones EC, Horsburgh MJ, Foster SJ, Vogel SN, et al. Selective roles for Toll-like receptor (TLR)2 and TLR4 in the regulation of neutrophil activation and life span. Journal of Immunology. 2003;**170**:5268-5275. DOI: 10.4049/jimmunol.170.10.5268

[80] Takehara M, Seike S, Sonobe Y, Bandou H, Yokoyama S, Takagishi T, et al. Clostridium perfringens α-toxin impairs granulocyte colony-stimulating factor receptor-mediated granulocyte production while triggering septic shock. Communications Biology. 2019;**2**:1-12. DOI: 10.1038/s42003-019-0280-2

[81] Hayashi F, Means TK, Luster AD. Toll-like receptors stimulate human neutrophil function. Blood. 2003;**102**:2660-2669. DOI: 10.1182/blood-2003-04-1078

[82] Sadeghi K, Wisgrill L, Wessely I, Diesner SC, Schuller S, Dürr C, et al. GM-CSF down-regulates TLR expression via the transcription factor PU.1 in human monocytes. PLoS One. 2016;**11**:e0162667. DOI: 10.1371/journal.pone.0162667

[83] Meisel H, Bockelmann W. Bioactive peptides encrypted in milk proteins: Proteolytic activation and thropho-functional properties. In: van Leeuwenhoek A editor. Int. J. Gen. Mol. Microbiol, 1999. pp. 207-215. DOI: 10.1023/A:1002063805780

[84] Millon L, Manteaux A, Reboux G, Drobacheff C, Monod M, Barale T, et al. Fluconazole-resistant recurrent oral candidiasis in human immunodeficiency virus-positive patients: Persistence of Candida albicans strains with the same genotype. Journal of Clinical Microbiology. 1994;**32**:1115-1118. Available from: http://www.ncbi.nlm.nih.gov/pubmed/8027327 [Accessed: 31 January 2020]

[85] Popa LG, Popa MI, Mihai IR. Case-control study to evaluate the link between immunosuppression and Candida spp. infection. Roumanian Archives of Microbiology and Immunology. 2005;**64**:72-76

Section 4

Breast Feeding: Microbiological Aspects

Chapter 6

Prophylactic and Therapeutic Role of Human Breast Milk Proteins and Bioactive Peptides against Neonatal Bacterial Infections

Sandeep Kaur, Mandeep Kaur Panaich, Simrat Kaur Virk, Mahima Choudhary, Chandni Sharma, Sunita Chauhan, Parul Chadha and Vandana Sharma

Abstract

Breast milk represents nature's best mechanism to provide complete nourishment and protection to the newborn. Human breast milk acts as a store house of an array of bioactive factors, which includes antimicrobial proteins and antimicrobial peptides that confer early protection while lowering the incidence of developing various infections and exhibiting immune modulation property to activate the immune cells to fight against the invading pathogens. Among the bioactive peptides, endogenous peptides present in breast milk have opened a new window of research on studying their unique mechanisms of action. This will help in incorporating these peptides in formula milk for meeting special needs where breastfeeding is not possible. The present chapter aims to give a deep insight into the various antimicrobial peptides and the newly reported endogenous peptides in human breast milk with emphasis on their levels and activity in preterm milk as data related to this is lacking and preterm newborns are highly vulnerable to acquire infections. Further, the chapter focuses on highlighting the antibacterial mechanisms adopted by the bioactive peptides for protection against the neonatal bacterial pathogens with special emphasis on the infections caused by resistant bacterial strains in hospital settings (neonatal wards) and their future implications.

Keywords: breast milk, neonatal infections, antimicrobial proteins, antimicrobial peptides, preterm, necrotizing Enterocolitis

1. Introduction

Breastfeeding provides a nursing infant with a plethora of bioactive molecules evolved to optimally develop the infants overall health. Traditionally breast milk was considered to serve only as a source of nutrition but breast milk is actually a perfect store house of an array of bioactive molecules essential for the overall development and protection of the newborn. It is considered as the best functional food for all instances, whether preterm or full term that is produced specifically by each mother to satisfy her unique infant. World Health Organization (WHO) recommends exclusive breastfeeding until 6 months and continuation of breastfeeding until 2 years as part of mixed diet [1, 2]. Past studies clearly indicate that as compared to formula fed infants, breast fed infants present lower incidence of microbial infections, better quality and composition of their gut flora, better cognitive functions, reduced risk of allergy with a stronger immunity to fight against infections in their future as well [3–6].

These properties and benefits of breastfeeding are due to the presence of multitude of bioactive molecules in human breast milk that help to protect the newborn from pathogenic microbes while strengthening infant's immune system. Among the major bioactive molecules are the milk proteins present. Colostrum has high concentration of proteins, is low in fat and carbohydrates than mature milk indicating that its primary purpose is to provide immediately as many bioactive proteins and peptides to the newborn aimed for its protection against microbial insult [7, 8].

These bioactive proteins serve various physiological functions which include enhancement of nutrient absorption by specific binding proteins facilitating the uptake of nutrients, assistant in digestion and growth stimulation. One of the major role of bioactive proteins is their antimicrobial effect as these molecules have broad spectrum antimicrobial activity in vitro against bacteria, viruses, and fungi, as well as synergistic activity with conventional antibiotics [9–11].

Antimicrobial proteins are multifunctional defense molecules that are highly concentrated in early lactation and decrease with progressing lactation. Their composition in milk changes to serve to the growing and changing needs of infant. They present a strong defense against the pathogens thus protecting the highly vulnerable infant while its immune system is still being developed. Antimicrobial proteins (**AMPrs**) and antimicrobial peptides (**AMPs**) exhibit their effect through many different mechanism and unique ways. They are involved in (a) direct outright killing the microbes, (b) neutralizing the bacteria and viruses and making them ineffective or (c) indirectly by blocking the initial attachment/adherence of the bacteria to mucosal surfaces. Besides this, these molecules also modulate the immune system by activating immune cells against infectious agents and strengthening the innate system against life-threatening infections and those targeting the mucosal lining (gastrointestinal infections, skin infections, respiratory tract infections) [12–14]. The combination of immunomodulation and antimicrobial factors help the child to avoid the development of various childhood infections and inflammatory diseases. Another major role played by breast milk proteins is the development of infant's gut flora exerted due to the prebiotic effect [10, 15]. Therefore, breast milk is a unique and complex reservoir of multitude of proteins and peptides all of which work in a synergistic manner to maximize the benefits in favor of the growing infant.

Another area of interest pertains to endogenous peptides present in human milk and their unique role that still warrants further research. These peptides are derived from proteins by specific proteases, many possess antibacterial action [16, 17]. Studying such endogenous peptides especially their role in preterm milk is of paramount importance in developing functional foods to cater to the special need of low birth weight infants (LBW) as well as preterm infants that stand at a higher chance of developing infections than term infants.

The role of milk derived antimicrobial proteins and peptides against neonatal pathogens and their clinical utility is definitely a complex topic and needs more detailed investigation. The present chapter focuses on various bioactive proteins and peptides involved, their mechanisms, spectrum of activity against range of bacterial infections with special emphasis on preterm infants and role of these molecules against resistant infections that are on rise in neonatal wards. Finally, future implications pertaining to use of newer technologies to exploit various human milk derived proteins and novel peptides as therapeutic and preventive intervention strategy has been highlighted.

2. The human milk proteome

Human breast milk is an ideal nutrition to the infants consisting of 87% water, 1% protein, 4% lipid and 7% carbohydrate along with various minerals and vitamins [15]. These bio-components of breast milk have been shown to provide bioactivities that are important for infant growth and development. The largest variety of bioactivities, however, is provided by proteins in breast milk [18].

Breast milk contains a wide array of proteins which are present in the form of enzymes/proteases, glycoproteins, and endogenous peptides. They provide unique biological activities, ranging from antimicrobial effects to immunostimulatory functions, facilitating the digestion and uptake of other nutrients in the milk such as iron, calcium and vitamin B besides providing sufficient amounts of essential amino acids to breast-fed infants [8]. The concentration and composition of human milk proteome changes continuously in their composition and concentration throughout gestational age and lactation stage. Over the last several years, an extensive analysis of the protein composition of term and preterm breast milk has been done [19–21]. Results indicate both quantitative as well as qualitative modifications through lactation in both term and preterm breast milk. Breast milk obtained from mothers who deliver preterm showed significantly higher protein content than that of mothers who deliver at term [22, 23]. The mean total protein content in preterm milk has been reported to range from 3.0 to 1.9 g/dl, and in term milk to vary from 2.2 to 1.1 g/dl over the first 4 weeks postpartum [19, 20, 24–26]. As lactation stage proceeds from colostrum to transitional milk, a gradual and physiological decrease in protein quantity occurs in both kinds of milk [26–28]. A decrease of protein levels by 30% was reported in preterm milk and by 50% in term milk from the first to eighth weeks of lactation [20, 29]. The concentration of proteins remains relatively constant thereafter in mature (term) milk. However, according to Lucas and Hudson [30], the volume of milk produced is an important determinant of protein content. They negatively correlated the postnatal age of the donor with milk protein concentration. Also, for feeding preterm infants, the lower level of total protein and specific amino acids from donor (typically, term, late lactation) milk alone is limiting, and requires additional supplementation. Many other factors also influence the protein content of human term milk. Bachour et al. [31] showed that smoking and mother's basal metabolic index (BMI) and lactation stage significantly decreased the protein content (12%) of the term milk. Overweight mothers also showed a lower milk protein concentrations [32]. The treatment of expressed milk also induces changes in the valuable nutrients contained in human milk. Ramirez-Santana et al. [33] evaluated the effect of cooling storage at 4°C and freezing storage at −20°C and −80°C on bioactive factors in human colostrum. The results interpreted that colostrum can be stored at 4°C for up to 48 h or at −20°C or −80°C for at least 6 months without losing its immunological properties provided by bioactive proteins. Similar study reported that lactating mother can pump the milk and refrigerate it for later consumption without compromising on the antibacterial potency of their milk against for up to 24 h [34].

Bjorksten et al. [35] and Evans et al. [36] reported no significant changes in human term milk proteins after freezing for 3 months. Another study suggested that frozen storage resulted in a lower reduction in various bioactive proteins as compare to pasteurization in term milk [37] Similarly, Chang et al. [38] revealed a non-significant decrease in most of the bioactive proteins in frozen as well as in low-grade heat treated (below 60°C) term milk. They proposed frozen breast milk as an alternative choice if fresh breast milk is unavailable. The Academy of Breastfeeding Medicine has a protocol for home storage of human milk that can be used to guide mothers in these activities to optimize the integrity of expressed and stored milk.

3. Breast milk and antimicrobial proteins

Human milk possesses inherent antimicrobial proteins that have been attributed to the defense against number of pathogens preventing their proliferation and invasion. The major antimicrobial proteins (AMPr) present in human milk act as first line of innate defense and are discussed below:

3.1 Lactoferrin

Human lactoferrin (HmLf) a multifunctional whey class of globular glycoprotein, found in abundance in human milk. The concentration is highest in colostrum at 5.5 g/L and decreases between 1.5 and 3.0 g/L in mature milk depending on the stage of lactation [39]. The decline in lactoferrin concentration is slower in preterm mother's milk than in full-term mother's milk [40]. Lactoferrin is an antiviral, antibacterial and anti-inflammatory protein. HmLF exert antimicrobial activity against Gram-positive [41–44] bacteria by either iron-depletion and/or disruption of bacterial membrane [45]. Lactoferrin also possesses anti-inflammatory properties and seems to be involved in phagocytic killing and immune responses [46]. The presence of human lactoferrin in breast fed infants indicate that it survive proteolytic digestion. Higher concentration found in the feces of premature infants suggests that these proteins play an active role in the infant gut [47].

3.2 Secretory immunoglobulin A (sIgA)

sIgA is the major immunoglobulin belonging to whey group of proteins present in human milk. The average concentration ranges from 2.0 g/L in colostrum to approximately 0.5 g/L in mature milk [48]. The secretory component works as a defense mechanism for the antibody molecules, protecting them from gastric acid and digestive enzymes, hence, resist digestion [49]. As a result, sIgA molecules remain active throughout the infants' gastrointestinal tract and protect against bacterial infections especially diarrheal diseases which are a major cause of morbidity and mortality in children in developing countries [50]. sIgA bind to pathogenic bacteria, toxins and other antigenic materials, such as lipopolysaccharide (LPS), thus, preventing their adherence and penetration into the intestinal epithelium without triggering inflammatory reactions that could be harmful to the newborn. This mechanism is called immune exclusion.

Apart from direct binding, sIgA can agglutinate bacteria non-specifically through oligosaccharide α-side chains of the immunoglobulin molecule. These oligosaccharides bind to fimbrial lectins, e.g., of *E. coli* and other bacteria [51]. Purified sIgA from human milk has been shown to protect the breast-fed infant by inhibiting the adhesion of enteropathogenic *Escherichia coli* (EPEC) to HEp- 2 cells in cell culture [52]. Another study demonstrated the ability of human milk sIgA to block the adhesion of *Staphylococcus aureus* strain in tissue culture.

3.3 Lysozyme

This protein constitutes a major fraction of the whey protein of breast milk. It is present in higher amounts in colostrum (0.36 g/L) and its concentration is slightly reduced in mature milk to 0.30 g/L [53]. Lysozyme is a protein that can exerts its antibacterial effect against gram positive bacteria independently by cleaving the 1–4 linkage between N-acetyl glucosamine and N-acetylmuramic acid in their cell wall. It may also act in concert with lactoferrin to kill both gram-positive and gram-negative bacteria and perhaps also against viruses. Electron microscopic studies showed that lactoferrin first binds to LPS in outer membrane of the bacteria creating holes through which lysozyme can penetrate and degrade the inner peptidoglycan matrix [8]. It is found intact in the stool of infant showing that it may exert its activity in the gut of breast fed infant.

3.4 κ-Casein (κ-CN)

k-casein, a small subunit of casein present in breast milk, is a highly glycosylated (90%) oligosaccharide. Concentration of kappa casein in colostrum is 25 and 1 g/L in mature milk [54]. The antimicrobial properties of the κ-casein portion of human milk fluids were first reported by Aniansson et al. [55]. κ-casein was showed to inhibit the adherence of *Streptococcus pneumoniae* to human respiratory tract epithelial cells in vitro. κ-casein prevents the attachment of bacteria to the mucosal lining as their oligosaccharides act as a receptor analogue having structures similar to exposed glycans on mucosal surface [56]. Others have demonstrated an inhibitory effect of κ-CN on the adhesion of *Helicobacter pylori* to human gastric mucous cells [57]. These studies clearly established that the actual anti-infective agent responsible for preventing infection in their respective cell types was the carbohydrate portion of the glycoprotein. Later, the fucose carbohydrate moiety was specifically identified as the primary factor responsible for inhibiting adhesion. Studies have also indicated that κ-CN in milk works together in a synergistic approach with lactoferrin, and sIgA work to protect the new born against microbial attack.

3.5 Osteopontin (OPN)

It is a multifunctional glycosylated and heavily phosphorylated acidic protein initially discovered in bones. With high variability among mothers and stages of lactation, the average concentration of osteopontin in breast milk is approximately (138 $\pm$ 79 mg/L, mean $\pm$ SD) [58]. Present in low concentration in colostrum but after 3 days of lactation, high levels are established. The levels decrease with advancing lactation, but about half maximal levels are maintained beyond 1 year of lactation [59]. In vitro experiments have indicated that human and bovine milk OPN are in part resistant to proteolysis in the infant intestinal tract, which makes OPN a potentially bioactive component of human milk [60]. It also plays an important role in immune activation and immune regulation by acting as chemotactic agent and stimulates both pro- and anti-inflammatory processes. It enhances B lymphocyte immunoglobulin production and proliferation and also influences cell-mediated immunity by inducing Th1 cells [61]. Furthermore, it also has been shown to form complexes with lactoferrin and act as carrier for other immunomodulator protein to enhance their competencies [62].

3.6 Haptocorrin

Haptocorrin is a heavily glycosylated protein present at a concentration of 5 mg/ml in colostrum and 3 mg/ml matured milk. Haptocorrin is a vitamin B12-binding protein, stable against proteolytic digestive enzymes [46]. As the infants lack intrinsic factor required for absorption of vitamin B12, hence, haptocorrin may facilitate vitamin B12 absorption [63]. Even at low concentration, haptocorrin has been shown to possess antibacterial activity against pathogenic strains of *E. coli* and thus may serve as a defense protein against *E. coli* related infection [64]. However, more studies delineating the effect of the bacterial strain and it's mode of action is required as its antimicrobial role has been shown to be limited to very few pathogens.

3.7 Lactoperoxidase

A member of whey protein, lactoperoxidase is secreted by mammary glands and is persistently present during lactation with concentration of 1–1.5 units/ml [65]. Lactoperoxidase is a glycoprotein and it is resistant to proteolysis [66], thus playing a role in infant host defense. It forms lactoperoxidase system with thiocyanate (SCN^-) present naturally in human milk, and H_2O_2, which is generated by bacteria [67]. In the presence of H_2O_2, lactoperoxidase oxidases SCN^- to hypothiocyanite ($OSCN^-$), which has antimicrobial activity against both Gram positive and Gram negative bacteria [68]. These chemical reactions also cause leakage of potassium ions, amino acids, and peptides across the damaged cytoplasmic membrane. Lactoperoxidase together with sIg and lysozyme help to eradicate microorganisms from the small intestine without inflammation, contributing to the development of a healthy microbiome [69].

3.8 α-Lactalbumin

The most well characterized and primary whey protein in human milk is α-lactalbumin [70, 71], which accounts for 20–25% of total breast milk proteins. During its digestion, peptides appear to be transiently formed that have antibacterial and immunostimulatory properties, thereby possibly help in providing protection against infection. Various hydrolytic products of α-lactalbumin have shown antimicrobial activity against *E. coli*, *Klebsiella pneumoniae*, *Staphylococcus*, *Streptococcus*, and *C. albicans* [72].

3.9 Mucins

Mucins are high molecular mass glycoproteins (200–2000 kDa) heavily glyosylated proteins with variable number of tandem repeats, i.e., mucin domains [73]. Mucins are found within the milk fat globule membranes (MFGM), and typically make up less than 1% of total protein. At least 16 mucins have been identified in humans. Mucin-1 and Mucin-4 have been identified as the major human milk mucins [73]. Mucins provide protection against gastrointestinal and respiratory tracts infections by decreasing the adhesion of pathogens to the cell surface. Mucin-1 specifically has been reported to inhibit the invasion of *Salmonella typhimurium*, in a model of fetal intestinal cells, at concentrations that are similar to that of human milk [73]. Sialic acid moiety of mucin-1 interacts with pathogen thereby inhibiting the ability of the pathogen to bind to its infant host cell surface glycan receptor.

3.10 Lactadherin (milk fat globular membrane protein; MFGMP)

Lactadherin is a 46 kDa mucin associated sialyated glycoprotein found in milk fat globule membrane. In a study reported by Newburg et al. [74], 200 infants in Mexico City from birth to 2 years of age were closely monitored for rotavirus infection symptoms. Milk samples were obtained from the respective mothers weekly until 4 weeks post-partum. The milk samples were taken immediately before an infant's episode of rotavirus infection and levels of lactadherin, butyrophilin, mucin, and secretory IgA were determined. Results indicated that concentration of lactadherin in the milk samples fed to infants belonging to asymptomatic group was 48.4 (range 5.6–180) μg/mL while in the symptomatic group, it was lower, i.e., 29.2 (6.2–103.4) μg/mL. No such association between symptom status and concentrations of butyrophilin, mucin, or secretory IgA was found. These findings indicated that Lactadherin concentrations showed a significant association with symptoms in rotavirus-infected breastfed infants and is representative of a class of non-antibody glycoconjugates in human milk having protective effect against symptomatic rotavirus infection.

4. Breast milk: reservoir of antimicrobial peptides (AMPs)

Human milk derived bioactive peptides are low-density molecules (5–90 amino acids) exhibiting their bioactivity features when separated from the parental proteins. These human milk peptides not only act as sources of amino acids, but they are also involved in immune-modulation, opioid-like activity, antioxidant, antimicrobial, and antiviral action, and probiotic action. These peptides when released may express activity different from that of the parent protein. This may account for their "encrypted" role other than parent protein after digestion [75]. Nielsen et al. [76] identified a total of 5264 unique peptides by mass spectrometry deriving from human and bovine milk proteins. Of these 1722 and 3399 originated from bovine and human milk proteins, respectively. β-casein accounted for 71.2% of the total human peptide ion intensity, with αs1-casein and κ-casein combining for an additional 11.7%.

Anti-microbial peptides (AMPs) exhibit activity against an array of neonatal pathogens both Gram positive (*Staphylococcus aureus*, *Streptococcus pneumoniae*, Group B Streptococcus, i.e., GBS) and Gram negative bacteria (*E. coli*, *Klebsiella pneumoniae*), mycobacteria, fungi and even the viruses [14, 77–79]. AMPs are expressed either constitutively or their expression can be inducible in response to certain pro-inflammatory stimuli. AMPs are cationic peptides that destroy bacteria in a unique way that is less prone to resistance. They initially target the bacteria via electrostatic contact at the anionic bacterial surface, i.e., AMPs interact with the highly negatively charged surface of the membrane consisting of lipopolysaccharide. This is then followed by self-promoted uptake while the AMPs insert and translocate to the outer bilayer to bind the anionic inner membrane [80]. This leads to rapid killing and lysis due to serious reduction of membrane integrity at high concentrations with some AMPs, also having intracellular targets such as DNA [81]. The concept of extracellular entrapment of bacteria by AMPs at epithelial surfaces and within the bloodstream is also one mechanism.

Although many AMPs of bovine origin have been studies in detail, but we are focused on detailing the antimicrobial peptides of human origin and their mode of action. Studying the activity and properties of human origin antimicrobial peptides will open a new window of alternate therapy targeting the treatment of infections resilient to the action of antibiotics especially in neonatal scenario. Also, such potent peptides can be further isolated, cloned and purified to be incorporated into infant formula feed acting as a ready therapy given through food to the highly vulnerable preterm infants. The major antimicrobial peptides present in human milk and their mechanism of action (**Figure 1**) reported till date are as follows.

4.1 Defensins

Defensins (2–6 K Da) are small cysteine rich cationic proteins that participate as host defense peptides against bacteria, fungi and enveloped/non enveloped viruses. Defensins can be categorized broadly as α-defensins, β-defesins and ϴ-defensins. α-defensins are produced in neutrophils and NK cells mostly in a constitutive manner whereas β-defensins are secreted by epithelial cells of various kinds which also include mammary gland. Armogida et al. [82] identified expression of hbd-2 gene in 15% of mammary epithelia cells. Baricelli et al. [83] quantified human β-defensins-2 (HBD-2) levels in colostrum and mature milk from 100 donors. The colostrum showed concentration ranging from 2.5 to 16.3 μg/ml whereas mature milk showed a low concentration of an average of 0.97 μg/ml.

They also reported that HBD-2 had potent activity against three opportunistic pathogens *Salmonella*, *E. coli* and *Pseudomonas aeruginosa*. It also showed activity of 4 *μg/ml against multi-drug resistant Acinetobacter baumanii*. These molecules have been shown to form nets to trap bacteria and combat invasion into deeper tissue [84]. These findings highlight the protective role of this peptide against serious gastrointestinal infections in neonatal population.

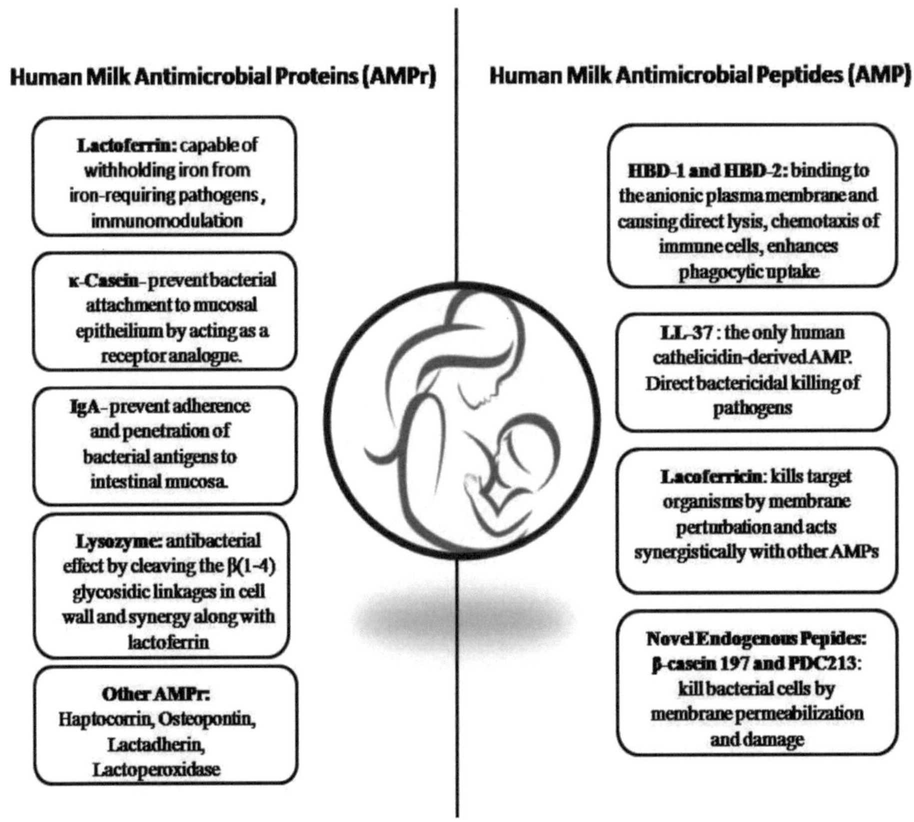

Figure 1.
Summary of different antimicrobial proteins and peptides in human Milk and their action.

Jia et al. [85] studied the levels of human β-defensins-1 (HBD-1) in human breast milk by western immunoblotting and reverse HPLC. They detected that level of HBD-1 was 1–10 μg/ml in mature milk and exhibited antimicrobial activity against *Escherichia coli*. In other study, breast tissue sampled from lactating mothers also showed hBD-1 mRNA expression in mammary gland epithelial cells and in active milk [86]. HBD1 also showed killing activity against *E. coli* at a conc. of 5 μg/ml and against *Salmonella enteritidis* through formation of entrapping nets in a redox dependent mode of action [87]. HBD-1 may act synergistically with other peptides present in breast milk. Also, HBD-1 acts as a chemotactic agent to recruit dendritic cells, T-cells to mucosal surfaces (respiratory, gastrointestinal, and nasopharynx) thus acting as a link between innate and adaptive immunity for the neonate [88].

4.2 Cathelicidins

Cathelicidins are multifunctional bactericidal peptides characterized by a highly conserved N-terminal domain of about 100 amino acid residues. This 14 kDa cathelin-like domain is flanked by a signal peptide domain (approximately 30 residues long) on its N-terminus, and by an antimicrobial peptide region on its C-terminus. The single 16 kDa human cathelicidin is denoted as hCAP18 and it becomes active only upon proteolytic cleavage into cathelin domain and cathelicidin-derived AMP yielding LL-37 [89]. This LL-37 is the only human cathelicidin-derived AMP secreted by mammary gland and present in human milk [90].

Human cathelicidin hCAP18/LL-37 mRNA expression was confirmed in human milk cells showing an increase in expression levels at 30 and 60 days after parturition. Further, western blot analysis showed that LL-37 was secreted and present in the mature peptide form in human milk and is present in expressed breast milk (EBM) of mothers of both term and preterm infants [91].

LL-37 exhibits antimicrobial activity against both Gram-positive and Gram-negative bacteria., The ability of cathelicidins and defensins to directly confer protection against bacterial colonization of epithelial surfaces has been shown in gut, lung, and skin [92, 93]. Chen et al. [94] also showed synergistic effect of antibacterial agents' human beta-defensins, cathelicidin LL-37 and lysozyme against *Staphylococcus aureus* and *Escherichia coli*. Scheid et al. [95] examined antimicrobial activity of LL-37 (15 μg/ml) in hirudin-anticoagulated preterm and term human cord blood against *Staphylococcus aureus*, *Staphylococcus epidermis* and *Candida albicans* by CFU assay. LL-37 enhanced the antibacterial/antifungal activity against all three pathogens in term blood and against *S. epidermidis* in preterm blood.

4.3 Lactoferricin

Although Lactoferrin is not readily digested and is found intact in stool sample of infants, it is digested partially to give a peptide called "Lactoferricin". This peptide is able to inhibit adherence of *Escherichia coli* to intestinal cells [96]. Lactoferricin is also active against clinical isolates of enterohemorrhagic *E. coli* 0157H:7 at concentrations significantly less than either the lactoferrin hydrolysate or lactoferrin, itself [97]. The mechanism involved in killing the target bacteria is through membrane perturbation and this peptide also acts synergistically with other proteins and antimicrobial agents [98]. In addition to Lactoferricin, the role of Lf (1–11) has also emerged in the recent past [99] as Lf(1–11) was demonstrated to be active against gram-positive bacteria (*Staphylococcus* spp. and *Streptococcus mitis*) as well as gram-negative bacteria (*Acinetobacter baumannii*, *Pseudomonas* spp., *Klebsiella* spp., and *E. coli*) [98, 100].

4.4 Novel endogenous antimicrobial peptides

- **β-casein 197:** Fu et al. [101] used tandem mass spectrometry (MS/MS) to identify the peptides in both term and preterm human milk, and identified a peptide derived from β-casein: a sequence (197–213) from human β-casein. It is a 17 amino acid (197–213) peptide fraction of β-casein that is a newly found endogenous peptide hydrolyzed human from β-casein. It exhibits potent bactericidal property against *E. coli*, *S. aureus*, *Yersinia* spp. but no activity was seen against *Bacillus subtilis* and *Klebsiella pneumoniae* by disk diffusion assay. Electron microscopy images of treated cells revealed leaky cytoplasm and bleb like structures indicating the β-casein 197 peptide killed cells by means of membrane permeabilization instead of DNA binding.

- **PDC213:** Sun et al. [102] reported another novel endogenous peptide from human milk called PDC213. PDC213 was derived from β-casein (213–266 amino acid residue). This endogenous peptide identified by the group exhibited potent antimicrobial activity against *S. aureus* and *Yersinia enterocolitica* using in vitro assays. Furthermore, the group also found that PDC213 can effectively permeabilize the bacterial membrane to cause direct damage to the bacteria.

5. Neonatal infections: a brief overview

The first 28 days of life, i.e., the neonatal period is the most crucial and the most vulnerable time for survival of newborn. It is reported that in 2018, 2.5 million children died in the first month of their life which means 7000 neonates die each day with one-third dying on the day of birth [103]. An estimated 16 million neonatal deaths occur annually due to infection representing 40% of all neonatal deaths which is a very high percentage. Among the infections, diarrhea, pneumonia, neonatal sepsis and malaria are the leading causes [104]. Despite recent advances in neonatal intensive care and current treatment interventions, the global burden of neonatal deaths due to infections is high and represents a challenge especially in developing and poorer countries. The leading neonatal infections that account for the greatest morbidity and mortality among neonatal population have been highlighted below and in **Table 1**.

5.1 Neonatal sepsis

Neonatal sepsis remains serious complication especially in preterm and VLBW infants. Globally the greatest burden of neonatal sepsis falls in low resource developing countries [105]. It is divided as early onset sepsis (EOS) that occurs in first week of life and late onset sepsis (LOS) occurring after 1 week acquired after birth. Group B streptococcus (GBS) remains the dominant cause of EOS with 20–33% mortality in premature infants [106, 107]. *E. coli* is the second most common cause isolated from such cases especially in VLBW infants [108, 109]. LOS is largely caused by organisms acquired in postnatal period in infants exposed to invasive procedures, tubings, devices etc. Coagulase negative Staphylococci (CoNS) has emerged as one of the most commonly isolated pathogen in VLBW infants (22–65%) of LOS infection [110, 111]. *S. aureus* is associated with 4–8% of such cases of LOS. The increased incidence of MRSA isolates from neonatal sepsis is a matter of concern as 25% of infants infected with MRSA die [112].

Neonatal infections	Etiological agents (Bacterial) involved
Early onset sepsis (EOS)	Dominant: Group B Stretococcus (GBS), *E. coli* Less common: *Str. pyogenes, Str. pneumoniae, Haemophilus influenzae*
Late onset sepsis (LOS)	Commonly isolated: Coagulase negative Staphylococci (CoNS), *S. aureus* Others: *Acinetobacter baumannii, Str. pneumoniae*
Early onset pneumonia (EOP)	*Str. pneumoniae* (25% of cases), Group B Streptococcus (GBS), *E. coli, Klebsiella* spp., *S. aureus*
Late onset pneumonia (LOP)	*S. aureus* (dominant cause), *Str. pyogenes, Str. pneumoniae, E. coli* (less common)
VAP	Methicillin sensitive *S. aureus* (MSSA) and Methicillin resistant *S. aureus* (MRSA), CoNS, *Streptococcus pneumoniae*
Necrotizing Enterocolitis (NEC)	Members of Enterobactericea (*E. coli*, Uropathgenic *E. coli* (UPEC), *Klebsiella pneumoniae*) *Pseudomonas aeruginosa*, Coagulase negative Staphlycocci (CoNS), MRSA, *Clostridium difficle*
Infantile diarrhea	ETEC, EPEC, *Shigella flexneri, Salmonella* spp.
Neonatal skin infections	*S. aureus, S. epidermidis*, CoNS, *Strep. pyogenes, Strep. pneumoniae*
Other infections (Otitis media, sinusitis, conjunctivitis, urinary tract infections)	*S. aureus, S. epidermidis, Str. pyogenes Str. pneumoniae*, Group B Streptococci (GBS) *Pseudmonas aeruginosa, E. coli, Klebsiella* spp.

Table 1.
Commonly encountered neonatal infections in preterm and term neonates along with their etiology.

Among Gram negative organisms, *E. coli* (20–31% of LOS cases), *Klebsiella pneumoniae*, *Pseudomonas* spp. are also isolated with worse outcomes and high mortality seen.

5.2 Necrotizing Enterocolitis (NEC)

NEC is a common gastrointestinal emergency among preterm and very low birth weight (VLBW) infants but rare in full term infants. Its exact pathology and mechanism still has to be clearly understood. Despite advanced care of preterm infants in Neonatal Intensive Care Units (NICU), NEC remains the leading cause of morbidity and mortality in this population. It is estimated that 1–5% of all NICU admissions and 5–10% of all VLBW (≤1500 g) are affected or at risk of developing NEC with about 30% of them unable to survive their first week itself [113].

In 80% cases of NEC with intestinal perforation, members of Enterobactericeae especially *E. coli*, *Klebsiella pneumoniae* were present in peritoneal fluid in 75% of cases, Coagulase negative Staphylococci (CoNS) in 14% of cases and anaerobes in 6%. Even cases of MRSA associated with few cases of NEC have emerged [114].

5.3 Neonatal pneumonia

It is estimated that pneumonia contributes to more than 1.2 million neonatal deaths and an unknown number of still births each year worldwide. Early onset pneumonia is acquired during labor/delivery and late onset pneumonia is acquired during postnatal period from colonization of endotracheal tubing, ventilator tubing, intravenous lines, from clinical staff and hospital staff after 48 hours or more of invasive mechanical ventilation [115]. The causative agents involved have been delineated in **Table 1**. *Streptococcus pneumoniae* and Group B streptococcus (GBS) are commonly encountered in early onset cases. Ventilator associated pneumonia (VAP) is on common rise as it has emerged as the second most reason for antibiotic intervention in NICU [116, 117] with *S. aureus* being the dominate cause due to its biofilm forming ability. Rising rates of resistance to common antibiotic means more fatality rates from neonatal pneumonia especially in poorer nations emphasizing on need to exploit alternative intervention strategies.

5.4 Infantile diarrhea

Diarrhea has been described as the leading cause of deaths due to infection in the neonatal period. It accounts for more than 10.5% of all deaths and despite efforts focused to reduce the related mortality, it still represents the main preventable cause of deaths in newborns and young children [118, 119]. The underlying cause may be due to bacterial, viral and parasitic origin. Enterotoxigenic *E. coli* (ETEC), Enteropathogenic *E. coli* (EPEC), *Shigella flexneri*, *Salmonella* spp. are all involved in different cases of bacterial diarrhea outbreaks more concentrated in slum areas.

In addition to this, other neonatal infections commonly encountered include conjunctivitis, skin infections (Bullous impetigo, skin abscess, scalded skin syndrome), Otitis media, urinary tract infections, etc.

6. Protective role of breast milk against neonatal infections

Early and exclusive breastfeeding is one of the most important intervention strategies to reduce the risk of developing serious bacterial infections and related infant mortality [119, 120]. The risk of non-viral diarrhea is higher for non-breast-fed infants in the first 4–6 months of their life. A recent meta-analysis suggested that infants who were breast-fed for >4 months showed a three times reduced frequency of developing severe respiratory tract infection as compared with infants who were not breast-fed [121]. In other studies, breast milk in protection against otitis media and urinary tract infections was reported [122, 123]. There is also an increased risk of mortality in children due to suboptimal or insufficient breastfeeding, which is responsible for 11.6% of total deaths of children under 5 years old [124]. Mother milk is also the best option for preterm and very low birth infants as studies indicate the over expression and increased level of range of functional peptides in preterm milk that may act as ready source of protection for the vulnerable infant. Preterm infants due to their low intake of breast milk volumes and associated proteins and peptides may be actually at higher risk of developing serious life threatening infections like NEC, late onset sepsis, pneumonia, etc. [75]. **Table 2** summarizes the finding of few of the important studies elucidating the protective role of breast milk against common neonatal infections.

The antimicrobial proteins and range of antimicrobial peptides present in breast milk act synergistically adopting multiple mechanisms to inhibit disease progression by the invading pathogen. Human milk proteins and their derived peptides have been discussed in Sections 3 and 4. Antimicrobial peptides released from any source including breast milk circulate in infants' blood stream and provide an ongoing source of low-level of non-specific immune defense against potential invasive pathogens. LL-37 along with bactericidal permeability increasing protein (BPI) has been shown to be present in higher levels in infant's blood suffering from acute blood stream infections. Also, LL-37 exhibits significant inhibitory activity against

Target infection	Reference	Objective and study design	Result	Final outcome
Neonatal sepsis	[125]	**Objective:** To investigate the protective efficacy of breastfeeding against neonatal sepsis high risk population in Lahore, Pakistan. **Study Design:** A case–control study where 42 cases of neonatal sepsis from hospital and 270 age matched controls acted as participants Exclusive breast feeding was as most babies were partially breast fed and a few given formula feed or animal milk.	In the partially breast fed group there were 19 cases and 253 controls while in the group given no breast milk there were 23 cases and 17 controls. Therefore, the incidence of breast feeding was less among the cases than the controls, with an odds ratio of 18.	Even partial breast feeding protects against neonatal sepsis in premature infants.
Neonatal pneumonia	[126]	**Objective**: To assess whether breast feeding protects young children against pneumonia and whether this protection varies with age. **Study Design:** A nested case control study in Brazil where 152 infants aged 28–364 days who had been admitted to hospital for pneumonia participated in the study.	Results indicated that the babies who were not being breast fed were 17 times more likely to be admitted with pneumonia as compared to breast fed infants and this risk was higher in the initial 3 months of infancy.	Breast feeding protects young children against pneumonia, especially in the first months of life.
Acute respiratory illness (ARI), pneumonia and diarrhea	[127]	**Objective:** To assess the potential role of exclusive breastfeeding in reducing the incidence of deaths due to acute respiratory infections (ARI) and diarrhea **Study Design:** A prospective observational study was conducted on a birth cohort of 1677 infants who were born in slum areas of Dhaka, Bangladesh and followed from birth to 12 months of age. On basis of verbal autopsy and a structured questionnaire, the mortality attributable to ARI and diarrhea was measured.	The overall risk of infant deaths from all causes was 2.23 fold higher in infants with no or poor breast feeding as compared with infants with exclusive breastfeeding while the risk of deaths due to ARI and diarrhea was still higher, i.e., 2.40- and 3.94-fold higher in no or partially breast fed babies.	Exclusive breastfeeding in the first few months of life significantly decreases onset of ARI and Diarrhea.
Lower respiratory tract illness	[128]	**Objective:** To examine breastfeeding and the risk of hospitalization for lower respiratory tract disease in healthy full-term infants with access to modern medical care. **Study:** It was a meta-analysis of 33 studies.	Result from this meta-analysis indicated that among the infants with severe respiratory tract illnesses resulting in hospitalizations, more than tripling of them were those who were not breastfed for the initial 4 months of their infancy.	Breast feeding decreases risk of lower respiratory illnesses.
NEC	[129]	**Objective**: To determine the association between human milk (HM) intake and risk of necrotizing enterocolitis (NEC) or death among infants (401–1000 g birth weight).	Results indicated 13.6% infants died and developed NEC after 14 days of their birth. However, after the initial 14 days, the	Dose dependent effect was evident between intake of human milk and reduction in risk of developing NEC and

Target infection	Reference	Objective and study design	Result	Final outcome
		Study Design: Analysis of 1272 infants in the National Institute of Child Health and Human Development Neonatal Network Glutamine Trial was performed to determine if increasing HM intake was associated with decreased risk of NEC or death.	incidence of NEC decreased by a factor of 0.83 with every 10% increase in the total intake of Human milk. Therefore, a strong dose association was seen with a decreased risk of NEC or death among infants who received 100% human milk as a proportion to total enteral intake.	related death after the first 2 weeks of life among VLBW infants.
Ventilator-associated pneumonia (VAP)	[130]	**Objective**: To explore the use of mothers' own milk (colostrums, transitional milk, and mature milk) as oral care in the ventilator-associated pneumonia (VAP)-prevention bundle of mechanically ventilated preterm infants weighing 1500 g or less. **Study Design:** Retrospective descriptive involving mechanically ventilated preterm infants weighing 1500 g or less admitted to a regional level III NICU in the Gulf South. To these, oral care with mothers' own milk was implemented as part of the VAP-prevention bundle and the outcomes that were assessed included rate of positive tracheal aspirates, positive blood cultures, the number of ventilator days, and length of stay.	Rates of positive tracheal aspirates and positive blood cultures showed reduced values in infants receiving oral care with mothers' own milk.	Use of mother's milk as part of oral care as VAP-prevention bundle is a feasible safe and effective practice and warrants further research.
Neonatal conjunctivitis	[131]	**Objective**: To investigate the effect of human breast milk (colostrums) in preventing neonatal conjunctivitis. **Study Design:** Randomized clinical trial where the intervention group with culture-negative eye swab received two drops of colostrum in each eye, antibiotic group received erythromycin ointment (0.5%), while control group received no treatment. All neonates were followed for the occurrence of clinical conjunctivitis for 28 days.	Results indicated that application of colostrum significantly decreases the onset of neonatal conjunctivitis in the test group as compared to control group ($p = 0.036$).	A positive effect with application of Human colostrums was found and thus can act as a favorable option in place of antibiotics against neonatal conjunctivitis.
NEC	[132]	**Objective**: To study the effects of feeding exclusively human milk (EHM) diet to premature infants on reducing the incidence of necrotizing enterocolitis (NEC) associated	In the control cohort, NEC onset after day 7 of life occurred in 15 of 443 infants (3.4%), significantly more than in the EHM cohort	Changing to an EHM milk diet through 33 weeks PMA reduced the incidence of NEC associated with enteral feeding.

Target infection	Reference	Objective and study design	Result	Final outcome
		with enteral feeding. **Study Design:** An observational study included all premature infants admitted to Level III NICU, at less than 33 weeks gestational age. An EHM diet was recommended which eliminated all bovine-based artificial milk, including bovine-based fortifier through the study period.	where NEC occurred in two of 199 infants (1%) ($p = 0.009$).	
NEC, LOS	[133]	**Objective**: To examine the effect of human milk on morbidity, specifically necrotizing enterocolitis (NEC), late onset sepsis (LOS), retinopathy of prematurity (ROP), bronchopulmonary dysplasia (BPD) and neurodevelopment in infants born ≤28 weeks' gestation. **Study Design:** Systematic review and meta-analysis where online databases were searched, and comparisons were grouped as follows: exclusive human milk (EHM) versus exclusive preterm formula (EPTF), any human milk (HM) versus EPTF, higher versus lower dose HM.	Human milk intake was associated with a clear protective effect against NEC, with a 4% reduction in incidence. Intake of exclusive human milk (EHM) in any volume was superior to intake of EPTF and the higher the dose the greater the protection.	Improving the intake of mother's own milk (MOM) and/or donor HM results in reducing the morbidity in this population.

Table 2.
Summary of some of the major studies focused on evaluating protective role of breast milk on outcome of various neonatal infections.

growth of *S. aureus* and *S. epidermidis*, two of the common pathogens involve in neonatal skin infections as well as cases of late-onset sepsis [134]. HBD-2 is the predominate defensin actively participating in reducing the incidence of respiratory infections and since preterm infants have lower levels of lung AMPs, they are unable to clear pathogens effectively [135]. Similarly, higher concentrations of HBD-2 appears to have a protective role once NEC pathology is established and in severe NEC. Low HBD-2 expression is a predisposing factor for developing NEC in preterm and low birth weight infants [136]. Low levels of defensins (HBD-1 and HBD-2) in preterm infants are associated with increased incidence of intestinal pathology and onset of NEC. Animal models have showed that depletion of Paneth cells rich in defensins followed by enteric infection in test animal resulted in a clinical picture akin to human NEC [137]. HBD-2 is directly involved in killing range of nosocomial pathogens (*E. coli, S. aureus, Klebsiella, Salmonella*) as showed by in vitro assays [138, 139].

Lactoferrin (LF) is a major contributor showing direct bactericidal action on range of neonatal pathogens. Murakami et al. [91] showed that 32 μM concentration of Lactoferrin was able to exhibit potent killing of 77% Group A Streptococcus (GAS), 40% *S. aureus* and 17% *E. coli*. Therefore, LF supplementation in VLBW infants is an ideal prophylactic treatment option for reducing the incidence of deaths and complication due to serious infections such as blood stream infections, infantile diarrhea, NEC in this population. These findings form the rationale for further exploiting the potential clinical utility of antimicrobial proteins and peptides in the prevention and treatment of infections in infants.

7. Preterm infants: a special case

Prematurity has been reported to be second most common cause of death in children under 5 years of age. Preterm infants are those born before 37 weeks of completed gestation, extremely preterm are those born at less than 28 weeks of completed gestation whereas very preterm refers to infants born between 28 and 32 weeks of gestation [140]. The incidence of premature birth and related deaths have been steadily increasing each year with an estimated 15 million babies born preterm [15]. Such infants are at increased risk of development of serious life threatening infections such as necrotizing enterocolitis (NEC), late onset sepsis (LOS), bloodstream infections, pneumonia and other complications.

Therefore, the challenge is to further improve the future of preterm infants with early protection to be given immediately after birth starting in the neonatal care units.

Maternal milk, a complex fluid with several bioactive proteins and peptides is beyond doubt the best option for the preterm infant [141]. Literature reveals that bioactive factors are found in much higher levels in preterm milk as compared to full-term milk and such factors are totally lacking in formula milk and significantly decreased in donated milk. This focuses on the use of human milk fortifiers containing the useful functional peptides as an ideal choice acting as a prophylactic supplement to protect the preterm infant where breastfeeding is unavailable or insufficient.

Preterm milk has higher protein and peptide levels as reported by past workers [75, 142]. Ferranti et al. [143] found more than 100 peptides originating by break-down of casein protein from mother who gave birth at 25 week gestation which is a case of extreme preterm delivery. Similarly, Armaforte et al. [144] also found via 2D-SDS page technique that low molecular weight casein fragments are over expressed in preterm milk as compared to term milk whereas intact αS1-casein and ß-casein were present in low concentrations in preterm milk than term milk. Similarly, Dallas and co-workers [145] reported that protein breakdown was higher with higher level of plasmin activity seen in preterm milk. This indicates higher protein degradation and higher release of endogenous and antimicrobial peptides in preterm milk. These findings clearly indicate that antimicrobial peptides present in higher amounts act as a ready source to fight off infection at different levels for the wellbeing and early life protection of the preterm infants while the infants own protein digestion ability is not fully developed while compensating for the underdeveloped innate system of these vulnerable preterm infants.

Ronayne et al. [146] studied the level of lactoferrin in term and preterm milk and observed that the levels of lactoferrin remained constant in preterm group from eight post-partum day onwards while the levels showed a significant decline in term milk. This indicates that high levels are very much required in maintaining protective barrier against pathogens in preterm infants. Albenzio et al. [147] also found while studying lactoferrin levels from 28 mothers belonging to term and preterm cases that highest values of lactoferrin were detected in preterm infant maternal milk from infants with low weight (less than 1400 g). These findings again point towards use of tailored supplementation strategies of Lactoferrin in neonatal units and even after home discharge. The newly isolated endogenous peptides mentioned earlier in Section 4.4, i.e., PDC213 and ß-casein-197 have also been reported to be present in significantly higher concentrations in preterm milk as compared to term milk samples suggesting the role of breast milk naturally tailored to aid in giving maximum protection to such infants.

Human milk peptides also play an important role in preventing the onset of serious infections in VLBW infants. Meinzen-Derr et al. [129] studied the association between total human milk intake and the risk of developing necrotizing enterocolitis (NEC), a common cause of early death in extremely low birth infants. After, analysis of 1272 infants in a multicenter randomized, double-blind trial, results demonstrated protective effect of human milk intake with a dose dependent relationship seen between milk intake volumes and risk of developing NEC or death in such low birth weight infants. Similar cohort study also reported significantly lower rates of sepsis and death in low birth infants receiving less than 50 ml per kg per day of fortified human milk [148]. Sisk et al. [149] also reported six-fold decrease in the odds of NEC among 202 very low birth infants that received at least 50% human milk intake. Trend et al. [150] recently investigated the levels and antimicrobial activity of antimicrobial proteins and peptides in breast milk consumed by preterm infants, and whether deficiencies of these factors were associated with late-onset neonatal sepsis (LOS). They collected breast milk from mothers of preterm infants (32 weeks gestation) was collected on days 7 (n = 88) and 21 (n = 77) postpartum and concentrations of lactoferrin, LL-37, HBD-1 and HBD-2 were measured. Results indicated that levels of most AMPs and antibacterial activity in preterm breast milk were higher at day 7 than at day 21. The consumption of AMPs was significantly lower in preterm infants who subsequently developed LOS compared to matched controls. This highlights the need for research to improve upon the total feed intake, i.e., feeding tolerance, feeding volumes or increasing the total quantity of milk AMPs consumed through supplementation, that may be useful in reducing the risk of LOS in preterm infants.

7.1 Human milk fortification for preterm protection

Human milk is beyond doubt the best option to be given to the preterm. Human breast milk has many important proteins and peptides totally absent or present in low levels in bovine milk. For example, lysozyme is 1000 times highly concentrated in human milk than cow's milk. Osteopontin which is essential in establishing immunity is 10 times more concentrated in human milk. Similarly, Lactoferrin is 20 times more concentrated in human milk and is an excellent antimicrobial agent along with bifidogenic properties [151]. As per WHO and American Academy of Pediatrics, pasteurized Human Donor Milk (HDM) is recommended as a second choice where mother's own milk is unavailable to the preterm infant [152]. However, pasteurization may reduce some of the important immune cells, bioactive proteins and functional peptides therefore research is now being focused on to fortify human milk to fulfill the need of the preterm infant. A randomized clinical trial reported that oral lactoferrin supplementation to preterm infants showed a decreased incidence of late-onset sepsis, a common cause of early deaths in such infants [153]. Enrichment of donated milk with essential disease fighting proteins and peptides to be given as soon as possible and until discharge from hospital is required for the preterm infant as recommended by European Society of Pediatric Gastroenterology, Hepatology and Nutrition [154]. Clinical study on bovine lactoferricin added to infant formula showed significant reduction in upper respiratory diseases in such infants aged 6–12 months of age [155].

Manzoni et al. [156] also reported a reduction in sepsis cases in premature infants which were given oral supplements of bovine lactoferricin. This opens a new window of use of supplementation of human lactoferrin based fortifiers acting as a therapy for the target infants.

Low birth weight infants may take very low volumes of mother's milk and due to these low volume intake, the levels of useful bioactive peptides may also be deficient in such infants. In such cases, human milk should be supplemented with external factors so that even low volumes carry enough of the protective peptides to meet the demand of the preterm and VLBW infants.

European milk Bank Association working group recognizes standard fortification as the most utilized regimen in NICU. It also encourages the concept of "Individualized Fortification" to optimize nutrient uptake further introducing the concept of "Adjustable Fortification" and "Target Fortification" to specifically modify the human milk to be administered to such infants [157]. However, we need to know more about the complexity of the various components of breast milk as there is a lot of variability in the levels and activity of different proteins and peptides from one mother to other and from one infant to other.

8. Breast milk in era of antibiotic resistance

Antimicrobial resistance is one of the leading global threat to public health worldwide. The VLBW and preterm infants admitted to NICU are at an increased risk of developing range of nosocomial infections and if such an infection is caused by a resistant strain, the situation becomes still worse to treat. Neonates are particularly at risk of exposure to resistant strains within the hospital environment that includes methicillin resistant *Staphylococcus aureus* (MRSA), Vancomycin resistant *S. aureus* (VRSA), methicillin resistant *Staphylococcus epidermidis*, penicillin resistant strains of *Streptococcus pneumoniae*, extended spectrum beta-lactamase producing *E. coli*, *Klebsiella pneumoniae*, etc. [158–160].

Mortality is higher for children with drug-resistant infections, such as MRSA (a common skin and soft tissue infection) and infections caused by extended spectrum beta-lactamase-producing bacteria [161]. It is estimated that sepsis infections due to resistant strains accounts for approximately 214,000 neonatal deaths each year [162]. There is an urgent need for development of novel antibacterial drugs with unique mechanism of action that are not susceptible to existing resistance mechanisms being adopted by the bugs.

Human milk proteins and peptides offer a potent solution to fight life threatening infections especially in the infant population. It has been postulated by many workers that bacterial resistance to antimicrobial proteins and peptides is much less likely to evolve than the conventional antibiotics owing to their broad non-specific antibacterial mechanism of action that include membrane disruption and inhibition of cellular proteases [163, 164]. Also, most of these proteins and peptides work in a

Study	Milk peptide involved	Major findings
[166]	Ranalexin	Ranalexin (belonging to cathelicidin class) along with lysostaphin combination found to rapidly kill MRSA strain without affecting skin normal flora.
[167]	Indolicidin and Ranalexin	A group designed four hybrid peptides (Indolicidin and Ranalexin) that exhibited strong antibacterial activity against MRSA in vitro.
[168]	Indolicidin	Indolicidin—another family of peptides belonging to cathelicidin alone as well in combination with antibiotic was able to clear MRSA biofilm.
[169]	LL-13 and LL-17 (truncated forms of LL-37)	LL-37 and its truncated forms (LL-13 and LL-17) alone or in combination with vancomycin showed that both the truncated forms showed significant synergy and increased the susceptibility of VRSA to vancomycin. These two peptides also showed a strong ability to inhibit in vitro MRSA biofilm formation.
[170]	LL-37	An in vitro and in vivo study of Nafcillin (b-lactam drug) identified that it enhances killing of MRSA by increasing the binding of LL-37 to the MRSA membrane.
[171]	LL-37 and IDR-1	LL-37 and IDR-1 (innate defense regulator peptide) useful in ameliorating MRSA induced pneumonia using in vivo model of pneumonia in C57Bl/6 mice. The peptide combination was able to restore pulmonary function and decrease release of inflammatory cytokines in vivo through their immunomodulatory effect.
[172]	Recombinant hCAP18/ LL-37	Reported prokaryotic expression of full length hCAP18/LL-37 and its cathelin like prosequence. The workers showed that human cathelin like domain acts as a cysteine proteinase inhibitor and showed potent in vitro activity against resistant strains of *E. coli* and MRSA.
[173]	Human lactoferrin	Study reported that the bacteriostatic activity of human lactoferrin is solely due to its iron-chelating binding properties and is not influenced by antibiotic resistance of the pathogen involved. Therefore, therapeutic approach based on the use lactoferrin combined is a potent therapy against infections caused by resistant strains.
[174]	Lactoferrin derived HLR1r -synthetic	Reported a novel antimicrobial peptide structurally derived from human milk protein lactoferrin, HLR1r. They demonstrated potent activity against MRSA using in vivo model of pig infected with MRSA. The peptide also exhibited anti-inflammatory properties with significant reduction in inflammatory cytokines (TNF-α, IL-6 etc.)
[175]	Recombinant Lactoferrin (rLF)	Studied the efficacy of novel recombinant mouse lactoferrin to protect MRSA infection in a mouse model of peritonitis. The protein exhibited unique immunomodulatory mechanism in ameliorating the infection by decreasing the levels of inflammatory cytokines (TNF-α, IL-6, IL-1β, IL-10) post lactoferrin treatment.

Table 3.
Summary of role of milk derived bioactive peptides activity against drug-resistant bacterial pathogens.

synergistic manner and thus work more efficiently in combination therapy. This also further decreases the frequency of developing of resistant mutants within the target population. Recent study at University of Helsinki examined 16 mother-infant pairs for antibiotic resistance patterns in the infant gut. The result showed that infants that are breastfed for at least 6 months have less antibiotic resistant bacteria in their gut as compared with babies fed for a shorter time [165]. The major studies focused on the evaluation of human milk derived proteins and/or peptides and their activity against resistant bacterial strains either in their purified form or in recombinant form are summarized in **Table 3**.

There is an urgent need for developing novel antibacterial drug with unique mechanisms of action that are not susceptible to existing resistant mechanisms. One such breakthrough discovery has been the purification of protein-lipid complex from human milk. Marks et al. [176] reported for the first time, the role of **HAMLET**, a novel protein-lipid complex purified from casein fraction of human milk. HAMLET stands for Human α-lactalbumin made lethal to tumor cells. This complex was able to kill both the resistant and sensitive strains of *Streptococcus pneumoniae*, leading cause of neonatal pneumonia and deaths [177]. Also, HAMLET complex when used along with common antibiotics (Penicillin, erythromycin, gentamycin) actually potentiated their effect as pneumococci was made more susceptible as demonstrated in vitro biofilm model and in vivo mice nasopharygeal colonization model. The complex also showed activity against resistant strains of *Haemophilus influenzae* and *Moraxella* spp. The protein complex binds to bacteria and stops the flow of ions in and out of the cells, it also blocks important enzymes required by the bacteria to obtain energy. This unique mechanism makes the bacterial cell weak and easily susceptible to damage by common antibiotics as HAMLET synergy reduced the dose of antibiotics by a factor of eight to kill MRSA, VRSA and *S. pneumoniae*. It was able to re-sensitize MRSA to methicillin and vancomycin intermediate *S. aureus* (VISA) to vancomycin by depolarization of bacterial membrane thus dissipating the Proton motive force leading to more access and easy binding of drug to target bacterial cell [178, 179].

9. Utility of human milk derived antimicrobial peptides and future implications

The potential role of various antimicrobial proteins and peptides present in breast milk against the large array of neonatal infections warrants serious future work towards decreasing neonatal morbidity and deaths by further exploiting their clinical utility.

Cellceutix Corporation has completed phase II trials of Brilacidin (synthetic analog of human defensin) in treating acute bacterial skin infections and preclinical testing against otitis media and ocular infections [78]. Lytix Biopharma has completed phase II trials of synthetic peptide, i.e., LTX-109 in impetigo (a problematic condition primarily affecting young children). Talactoferrin, a recombinant human LF, has been tested in a phase I study in preterm neonates [180]. Other AMPs, such as LF 1-11 (hLF1-11), have undergone safety and tolerability testing for delivery in healthy volunteers [181]. The use of recombinant congeners of AMPs represents an ideal treatment to improve circulating levels and thus improve outcomes from bacterial infection in infants especially in preterm infants. These peptides either induced endogenously or as exogenously administered congeners, may help prevent and treat infections in highly susceptible infants in early life. This is possible through production of recombinant human milk proteins in large quantities to be used for the manufacture of fortified infant formula for special cases. Ward et al.

[182] reported the production of commercial quantities of bioactive recombinant human lactoferrin in *Aspergillus awamori*. The technology combined with strain improvement program yielded high concentration of intact recombinant lactoferrin. Also, the use of transgenic animals as bioreactors for the synthesis of the recombinant proteins secreted into milk is worth exploring [183, 184]. With the advent of targeted genome editing technologies like CRISPR/Cas9 system, it has been possible to generate economically important animals that produce recombinant proteins in milk. Therefore, future strategies need to focus on isolation of unidentified novel milk peptides and their recombinant congeners for mass production that can be administered as supplementary feeds for prevention and treatment of the most devastating neonatal infections such as pneumonia, neonatal sepsis, diarrheal diseases, NEC, etc.

10. Conclusion

Human breast milk is the most powerful functional food known. It is a reservoir of bioactive proteins and peptides that contribute to the enormous health benefits of breast milk. Antimicrobial proteins and peptides present in breast milk confer protection against microbial insult. They play an active role against invasion by neonatal pathogens through direct and indirect mechanisms thus decreasing the associated neonatal morbidity and mortality. Further, these peptides are expressed at higher levels in preterm milk than term milk acting as ready source of protection for the preterm and VLBW infants. In the era of antibiotic resistance, the need to exploit these unique milk derived peptides become still more important as they represent an important alternative strategy to fight against drug resistant infections that is on the rise in the neonatal population as well. Research focusing on incorporation of novel antimicrobial proteins and peptides in formula feed or to be given along with donor milk may allow for providing early life protection to the preterm infants decreasing the incidence of premature deaths due to serious life threatening neonatal infections. The role of recombinant DNA technology for mass production of these novel antimicrobial peptides followed by their safety and efficacy trials warrants future work.

Conflict of interest

The authors declare no conflict of interest.

Author details

Sandeep Kaur[1], Mandeep Kaur Panaich[1], Simrat Kaur Virk[1], Mahima Choudhary[1], Chandni Sharma[1], Sunita Chauhan[1], Parul Chadha[2] and Vandana Sharma[1*]

1 Department of Food Science, Mehr Chand Mahajan DAV College for Women, Chandigarh, India

2 Department of Microbiology, Panjab University, Chandigarh, India

*Address all correspondence to: vandanamcm5@gmail.com

References

[1] The World Health Organization. Report of the Expert Consultation. The Optimal Duration of Exclusive Breast Feeding. Report Reference Number: WHO/NHD/01.09. Geneva, Switzerland. 2001. Available from: http://www.who.int/nutrition/publications/infantfeeding/WHO_NHD_01.09/en/ [Accessed: 30 January 2017]

[2] American Association of Pediatrics. AAP Reaffirms Breast Feeding Guidelines. 2012. Available from: https://www.aap.org/en-us/about-the-aap/aap-press-room/pages/aap-reaffirms-breast-feeding-guidelines.aspx [Accessed: 30 January 2017]

[3] Kramer MS, Aboud F, Mironova E, Vanilovich I, Platt RW, Matush L, et al. Breastfeeding and child cognitive development: New evidence from a large randomized trial. Archives of General Psychiatry. 2008;**65**(5):578-584. DOI: 10.1001/ archpsyc.65.5.578

[4] Dieterich CM, Felice JP, O'Sullivan E, Rasmussen KM. Breastfeeding and health outcomes for the mother-infant dyad. Pediatric Clinics of North America. 2013;**60**(1): 31-48. DOI: 10.1016/j.pcl.2012.09.010

[5] O'Sullivan A, Farver M, Smilowitz JT. The influence of early infant-feeding practices on the intestinal microbiome and body composition in infants. Nutrition and Metabolic Insights. 2015;**8** (Suppl 1):1-9. DOI: 10.4137/NMI.S29530

[6] Victora CG, Bahl R, Barros AJ, França GV, Horton S, Krasevec J, et al. Breastfeeding in the 21st century: Epidemiology, mechanisms, and lifelong effect. Lancet. 2016;**387**(10017): 475-490. DOI: 10.1016/S0140-6736(15) 01024-7

[7] Gao X, McMahon RJ, Woo JG, Davidson BS, Morrow AL, Zhang Q. Temporal changes in milk proteomes reveal developing milk functions. Journal of Proteome Research. 2012; **11**(7):3897-3907. DOI: 10.1021/ pr3004002

[8] Ballard O, Morrow AL. Human milk composition: Nutrients and bioactive factors. Pediatric Clinics of North America. 2013;**60**(1):49-74. DOI: 10.1016/j.pcl.2012.10.002

[9] Lonnerdal B. Bioactive proteins in human milk: Mechanisms of action. The Journal of Pediatrics. 2010;**156**(2 Suppl): S26-S30. DOI: 10.1016/j.jpeds.2009.11.017

[10] Lonnerdal B. Human Milk: Bioactive proteins/peptides and functional properties. Nestle Nutrition Institute Workshop Series. 2016;**86**:97-107. DOI: 10.1159/000442729

[11] Zhu J, Dingess KA. The functional power of the human milk proteome. Nutrients. 2019;**11**(8):1834. DOI: 10.3390/nu11081834

[12] Cacho NT, Lawrence RM. Innate immunity and breast milk. Frontiers in Immunology. 2017;**8**:584. DOI: 10.3389/ fimmu.2017.00584

[13] Lonnerdal B. Bioactive proteins in breast milk. Journal of Paediatrics and Child Health. 2013;**49**:1-7. DOI: 10.1111/ jpc.12104

[14] Hakansson AP. Protective effects of human milk antimicrobial peptides against bacterial infection. The Journal of Pediatrics. 2015;**91**:4-5. DOI: 10.1016/ j.jped.2014.10.001

[15] Boquien CY. Human milk: An ideal food for nutrition of preterm newborn. Frontiers in Pediatrics. 2018;**6**:295. DOI: 10.3389/fped.2018.00295

[16] Andreas NJ, Kampmann B, Mehring Le-Doare K. Human breast milk: A

review on its composition and bioactivity. Early Human Development. 2015;**91**:629-635. DOI: 10.1016/j.earlhumdev.2015.08.013

[17] Khaldi N, Vijayakumar V, Dallas DC, Guerrero A, Wickramasinghe S, Smilowitz JT, et al. Predicting the important enzymes in human breast milk digestion. Journal of Agricultural and Food Chemistry. 2014;**62**:7225-7232. DOI: 10.1021/jf405601e

[18] Lonnerdal B, Erdmann P, Thakkar SK, Sauser J, Destaillats F. Longitudinal evolution of true protein, amino acids and bioactive proteins in breast milk: A developmental perspective. The Journal of Nutritional Biochemistry. 2017;**41**:1-11. DOI: 10.1016/j.jnutbio.2016.06.001

[19] Atkinson SA. Effects of gestational stage at delivery on human milk components. In: Jenson RG, editor. Handbook of Milk Composition. New York, NY, USA: Academic Press Inc.; 1995. pp. 222-236

[20] Bauer J, Gerss J. Longitudinal analysis of macronutrients and minerals in human milk produced by mothers of preterm infants. Clinical Nutrition. 2011;**30**(2):215-220. DOI: 10.1016/j.clnu.2010.08.003

[21] Faerk J, Skafte L, Petersen S, Peitersen B, Michaelsen KF. Macronutrients in milk from mothers delivering preterm. Advances in Experimental Medicine and Biology. 2001;**501**:409-413. DOI: 10.1007/978-1-4615-1371-1_51

[22] Castellote C, Casillas R, Ramirez-Santana C, Perez-Cano FJ, Castell M, Moretones MG, et al. Premature delivery influences the immunological composition of colostrum and transitional and mature human milk. Journal of Nutrition. 2011;**141**(6):1181-1187. DOI: 10.3945/jn.110.133652

[23] Thibeau SM, D'Apolito K. Review of the relationships between maternal characteristics and preterm breast milk immune components. Biological Research for Nursing. 2012;**14**(2):207-216. DOI: 10.1177/1099800411400064

[24] Anderson DM, Williams FH, Merkatz RB, Schulman PK, Kerr DS, Pittard WB 3rd. Length of gestation and nutritional composition of human milk. The American Journal of Clinical Nutrition. 1983;**37**(5):810-814. DOI: 10.1093/ajcn/37.5.810

[25] Chandra RK. Immunoglobulin and protein levels in breast milk produced by mothers of preterm infants. Nutrition Research. 1982;**2**:27-30. DOI: 10.1016/S0271-5317(82)80023-7

[26] Gross SJ, Buckley RH, Wakil SS, McAllister DC, David RJ, Faix RG. Elevated IgA concentration in milk produced by mothers delivered of preterm infants. The Journal of Pediatrics. 1981;**99**(3):389-393. DOI: 10.1016/s0022-3476(81)80323-x

[27] Atkinson SA, Bryan MH, Anderson GH. Human milk: Difference in nitrogen concentration in milk from mothers of term and premature infants. The Journal of Pediatrics. 1978;**93**:67-69. DOI: 10.1016/S0022-3476(78)80602-7

[28] Lemons JA, Moye L, Hall D, Simmons M. Differences in the composition of preterm and term human mass index, and parity number of lipid, protein, and secretory immunoglobulin A concentrations of human milk. Breastfeeding Medicine. 1982;7:179-188

[29] Anderson GH, Atkinson SA, Bryan MH. Energy and macronutrient content of human milk during early lactation from mothers giving birth prematurely and at term. The American Journal of Clinical Nutrition. 1981;**34**(2):258-265. DOI: 10.1093/ajcn/34.2.258

[30] Lucas A, Hudson GJ. Preterm milk as a source of protein for low birthweight infants. Archives of Disease in Childhood. 1984;**59**(9):831-836. DOI: 10.1136/adc.59.9.831

[31] Bachour P, Yafawi R, Jaber F, Choueiri E, Abdel-Razzak Z. Effects of smoking, mother's age, body mass index, and parity number on lipid, protein, and secretory immunoglobulin A concentrations of human milk. Breastfeeding Medicine. 2012; **7**(3):179-188. DOI: 10.1089/bfm.2011.0038

[32] Nommsen-Rivers LA, Dewey KG. Growth of breastfed infants. Breastfeeding Medicine. 2009;**4** (Suppl 1):S45-S49. DOI: 10.1089/bfm.2009.0048

[33] Ramirez-Santana C, Perez-Cano FJ, Audi C, Castell M, Moretones MG, Lopez-Sabater MC, et al. Effects of cooling and freezing storage on the stability of bioactive factors in human colostrum. Journal of Dairy Science. 2012;**95**(5):2319-2325. DOI: 10.3168/jds.2011-5066

[34] Sharma V, Sharma C, Chauhan S, Kaur S. Effect of lactation age and storage on the antibacterial potency of human breast milk against neonatal pathogens. Journal of Pure and Applied Microbiology. 2018;**12**(3):1307-1314. DOI: 10.22207/JPAM.12.3.33

[35] Bjorksten B, Sepp E, Julge K, Voor T, Mikelsaar M. Allergy development and the intestinal microflora during the first year of life. The Journal of Allergy and Clinical Immunology. 2001;**108**(4):516-520. DOI: 10.1067/mai.2001.118130

[36] Evans TJ, Ryley HC, Neale LM, Dodge JA, Lewarne VM. Effect of storage and heat on antimicrobial proteins in human milk. Archives of Disease in Childhood. 1978;**53**(3): 239-241. DOI: 10.1136/adc.53.3.239

[37] Akinbi H, Meinzen-Derr J, Auer C, Ma Y, Pullum D, Kusano R, et al. Alterations in the host defense properties of human milk following prolonged storage or pasteurization. Journal of Pediatric Gastroenterology and Nutrition. 2010;**51**:347-352. DOI: 10.1097/MPG.0b013e3181e07f0a

[38] Chang JC, Chen CH, Fang LJ, Tsai CR, Chang YC, Wang TM. Influence of prolonged storage process, pasteurization, and heat treatment on biologically-active human milk proteins. Pediatrics and Neonatology. 2013;**54**(6): 360-366. DOI: 10.1016/j.pedneo.2013.03.018

[39] Lawrence RA, Lawrence RM. Breastfeeding: A Guide for the Medical Professions. 7th ed. Maryland Heights: Elsevier Mosby; 2011. p. 253

[40] Pandita A, Sharma D, Kumar C. Lactoferrin and its role in neonatology: A review article. Journal of Pediatrics & Neonatal Care. 2015;**2**:00062

[41] Bhimani RS, Vendrov Y, Furmanski P. Influence of lactoferrin feeding and injection against systemic staphylococcal infections in mice. Journal of Applied Microbiology. 1999; **86**(1):135-144. DOI: 10.1046/j.1365-2672.1999.00644.x

[42] Hendricks GM, Guo M. Bioactive components in human milk. In: Guo M, editor. Human Milk Biochemistry and Infant Formula Manufacturing. Cambridge, UK: Woodhead Publishing; 2014. pp. 33-54

[43] Farnaud S, Evans RW. Lactoferrin—A multifunctional protein with antimicrobial properties. Molecular Immunology. 2005;**40**(7):395-405. DOI: 10.1016/s0161-5890(03)00152-4

[44] Orsi N. The antimicrobial activity of lactoferrin: Current status and perspectives. BioMetals. 2004;**17**(3): 189-196. DOI: 10.1023/b:biom.0000027691.86757.e2

[45] Ellison RT III, Giehl TJ. Killing of gram-negative bacteria by lactoferrin and lysozyme. The Journal of Clinical Investigation. 1991;**88**:1080-1091

[46] Lonnerdal B, Iyer S. Lactoferrin: Molecular structure and biological function. Annual Review of Nutrition. 1995;**15**:93-110. DOI: 10.1146/annurev.nu.15.070195.000521

[47] Davidson LA, Donovan SM, Lonnerdal B, Atkinson SA. Excretion of human milk proteins by term and premature infants. In: Atkinson SA, Lonnerdal B, editors. Protein and Non-Protein Nitrogen in Human Milk. Boca Raton, FL: CRC Press; 1989. pp. 161-172

[48] Davidson GP. Passive protection against diarrheal disease. Journal of Pediatric Gastroenterology and Nutrition. 1996;**23**:207-212. DOI: 10.1097/00005176-199610000-00001

[49] Lawrence RA. Host-resistance factors and immunologic significance of human milk. Breastfeeding: A guide for the medical profession. Elsevier Health Sciences. 2005;**6**:171-214

[50] Goldblum RM. The role of IgA in local immune protection. Journal of Clinical Immunology. 1990;**10**:64

[51] Wold AE, Hanson LA. Defence factors in human milk. Current Opinion in Gastroenterology. 1994;**10**:652. DOI: 10.1016/s0022-3476(73)80453-6

[52] Delneri MT, Carbonare SB, Silva ML, Palmeira P, Carneiro-Sampaio MM. Inhibition of enteropathogenic *Escherichia coli* adhesion to HEp-2 cells by colostrum and milk from mothers delivering low-birth-weight neonates. European Journal of Pediatrics. 1997; **156**(6):493-498. DOI: 10.1007/s004310050646

[53] Haschke F, Haiden N, Thakkar SK. Nutritive and bioactive proteins in breastmilk. Annals of Nutrition & Metabolism. 2016;**69**(Suppl. 2):17-26. DOI: 10.1159/000452820

[54] Cuilliere ML, Trégoat V, Bene MC, Faure G, Montagne P. Changes in the kappa-casein and beta-casein concentrations in human milk during lactation. Journal of Clinical Laboratory Analysis. 1999;**13**(5):213-218. DOI: 10.1002/(SICI)1098-2825(1999)13:5<213::AID-JCLA4>3.0.CO;2-F

[55] Aniansson G, Andersson B, Lindstedt R, Svanborg C. Anti-adhesive activity of human casein against *Streptococcus pneumoniae* and *Haemophilus influenzae*. Microbial Pathogenesis. 1990;**8**:315-323. DOI: 10.1016/0882-4010(90)90090-d

[56] Newburg DS. Do the binding properties of oligosaccharides in milk protect human infants from gastrointestinal bacteria? The Journal of Nutrition. 1997;**127**:980S-984S. DOI: 10.1093/jn/127.5.980S

[57] Stromqvist M, Falk P, Bergstrom S, Hansson L, Lonnerdal B, Normark S, et al. Human milk kappa-casein and inhibition of *Helicobacter pylori* adhesion to human gastric mucosa. Journal of Pediatric Gastroenterology and Nutrition. 1995;**21**(3):288-296. DOI: 10.1097/00005176-199510000-00006

[58] Schack L, Lange A, Kelsen J, Agnholt J, Christensen B, Petersen TE, et al. Considerable variation in the concentration of osteopontin in human milk, bovine milk, and infant formulas. Journal of Dairy Science. 2009;**92**(11):5378-5385. DOI: 10.3168/jds.2009-2360

[59] Nagatomo T, Ohga S, Takada H, Nomura A, Hikino S, Imura M, et al. Microarray analysis of human milk cells: Persistent high expression of osteopontin during the lactation period. Clinical and Experimental Immunology. 2004;**138**(1):47-53

[60] Chatterton DEW, Rasmussen JT, Heegaard CW, Sørensen ES, Petersen TE. In vitro digestion of novel milk protein ingredients for use in infant formulas: Research on biological functions. Trends in Food Science and Technology. 2004;**15**:373-383. DOI: 10.1016/j.tifs.2003.12.004

[61] Wang KX, Denhardt DT. Osteopontin: Role in immune regulation and stress responses. Cytokine & Growth Factor Reviews. 2008;**19**: 333-345. DOI: 10.1016/j.cytogfr.2008.08.001

[62] Azuma N, Maeta A, Fukuchi K, Kanno C. A rapid method for purifying osteopontin from bovine milk and interaction between osteopontin and other milk proteins. International Dairy Journal. 2006;**16**:370-378. DOI: 10.1016/j.idairyj.2005.03.012

[63] Adkins Y, Lonnerdal B. Mechanisms of vitamin B12 absorption in breast-fed infants. Journal of Pediatric Gastroenterology and Nutrition. 2002; **35**:192-198. DOI: 10.1097/00005176-200208000-00016

[64] Adkins Y, Lonnerdal B. Potential host-defense role of a human milk vitamin B-12-binding protein, haptocorrin, in the gastrointestinal tract of breastfed infants, as assessed with porcine haptocorrin in vitro. The American Journal of Clinical Nutrition. 2003;**77**(5):1234-1240. DOI: 10.1093/ajcn/77.5.1234

[65] Shin K, Tomita M, Lonnerdal B. Identification of lactoperoxidase in mature human milk. The Journal of Nutritional Biochemistry. 2000;**11**: 94-102. DOI: 10.1016/s0955-2863(99)00082-0

[66] Kussendrager KD, van Hooijdonk AC. Lactoperoxidase: Physico-chemical properties, occurrence, mechanism of action and applications. The British Journal of Nutrition. 2000;**84**(Suppl 1):S19-S25. DOI: 10.1017/s0007114500002208

[67] Sharma S, Singh AK, Kaushik S, Sinha M, Singh RP, Sharma P, et al. Lactoperoxidase: Structural insights into the function, ligand binding and inhibition. International Journal of Biochemistry and Molecular Biology. 2013;**4**(3):108-128

[68] Sarr D, Toth E, Gingerich A, Rada B. Antimicrobial actions of dual oxidases and lactoperoxidase. Journal of Microbiology. 2018;**56**:373-386. DOI: 10.1007/s12275-018-7545-1

[69] Alexander DB, Iigo M, Yamauchi K, Suzui M, Tsuda H. Lactoferrin: An alternative view of its role in human biological fluids. Biochemistry and Cell Biology. 2012;**90**(3):279-306. DOI: 10.1139/o2012-013

[70] Lonnerdal B, Lien EL. Nutritional and physiologic significance of alpha-lactalbumin in infants. Nutrition Reviews. 2003;**61**:295-305. DOI: 10.1301/nr.2003.sept.295-305

[71] Permyakov EA, Berliner LJ. Alpha-lactalbumin: Structure and function. FEBS Letters. 2000;**473**:269-274. DOI: 10.1016/s0014-5793(00)01546-5

[72] Pellegrini A, Thomas U, Bramaz N, Hunziker P, von Fellenberg R. Isolation and identification of three bactericidal domains in the bovine α-lactalbumin molecule. Biochimica et Biophysica Acta. 1999;**1426**(3):439-448. DOI: 10.1016/s0304-4165(98)00165-2

[73] Liu B, Yu Z, Chen C, Kling DE, Newburg DS. Human milk mucin 1 and mucin 4 inhibit *Salmonella enterica* serovar Typhimurium invasion of human intestinal epithelial cells in vitro. The Journal of Nutrition. 2012;**142**(8): 1504-1509. DOI: 10.3945/jn.111.155614

[74] Newburg DS, Peterson JA, Ruiz-Palacios GM, Matson DO, Morrow AL,

Shults J, et al. Role of human-milk lactadherin in protection against symptomatic rotavirus infection. Lancet. 1998;**351**(9110):1160-1164. DOI: 10.1016/S0140-6736(97)10322-1

[75] Dallas DC, Guerrero A, Khaldi N, Borghese R, Bhandari A, Underwood MA, et al. A peptidomic analysis of human milk digestion in the infant stomach reveals protein-specific degradation patterns. The Journal of Nutrition. 2014;**144**(6):815-820. DOI: 10.3945/jn.113.185793

[76] Nielsen SD, Beverly RL, Underwood MA, Dallas DC. Release of functional peptides from mother's milk and fortifier proteins in the premature infant stomach. PLoS One. 2018;**13**(11): e0208204. DOI: 10.1371/journal.pone.0208204

[77] Hanson LA, Korotkova M. The role of breastfeeding in prevention of neonatal infection. Seminars in Neonatology. 2002;**7**(4):275-281. DOI: 10.1016/s1084-2756(02)90124-7

[78] Battersby AJ, Gibbons DL. The gut mucosal immune system in the neonatal period. Pediatric Allergy and Immunology. 2013;**24**(5):414-421. DOI: 10.1111/pai.12079

[79] Mohanty D, Jena R, Choudhury PK, Pattnaik R, Mohapatra S, Saini MR. Milk derived antimicrobial bioactive peptides: A review. International Journal of Food Properties. 2016;**19**: 837-846

[80] Wimley WC. Describing the mechanism of antimicrobial peptide action with the interfacial activity model. ACS Chemical Biology. 2010; **5**(10):905-917. DOI: 10.1021/cb1001558

[81] Le CF, Fang CM, Sekaran SD. Intracellular targeting mechanisms by antimicrobial peptides. Antimicrobial Agents and Chemotherapy. 2017;**61**(4): e02340-16. DOI: 10.1128/AAC.02340-16

[82] Armogida SA, Yannaras NM, Melton AL, Srivastava MD. Identification and quantification of innate immune system mediators in human breast milk. Allergy and Asthma Proceedings. 2004;**25**:297-304

[83] Baricelli J, Rocafull MA, Vazquez D, Bastidas B, Baez-Ramirez E, Thomas LE. β-Defensin-2 in breast milk displays a broad antimicrobial activity against pathogenic bacteria. The Journal of Pediatrics. 2015;**91**:36-43. DOI: 10.1016/j.jped.2014.05.006

[84] Chu H, Pazgier M, Jung G, Nuccio SP, Castillo PA, de Jong MF, et al. Human α-defensin 6 promotes mucosal innate immunity through self-assembled peptide nanonets. Science. 2012;**337**(6093):477-481. DOI: 10.1126/science.1218831

[85] Jia HP, Starner T, Ackermann M, Kirby P, Tack BF, McCray PB Jr. Abundant human beta-defensin-1 expression in milk and mammary gland epithelium. The Journal of Pediatrics. 2001;**138**(1):109-112. DOI: 10.1067/mpd.2001.109375

[86] Tunzi CR, Harper PA, Bar-Oz B, Valore EV, Semple JL, Watson-MacDonell J, et al. Beta-defensin expression in human mammary gland epithelia. Pediatric Research. 2000; **48**(1):30-35. DOI: 10.1203/00006450-200007000-00008

[87] Raschig J, Mailander-Sanchez D, Berscheid A, Berger J, Strömstedt AA, Courth LF, et al. Ubiquitously expressed Human Beta Defensin 1 (hBD1) forms bacteria-entrapping nets in a redox dependent mode of action. PLoS Pathogens. 2017;**13**(3):e1006261. DOI: 10.1371/journal.ppat.1006261

[88] Yang D, Chertov O, Oppenheim JJ. The role of mammalian antimicrobial peptides and proteins in awakening of innate host defenses and adaptive immunity. Cellular and Molecular Life

Sciences. 2001;**58**:978-989. DOI: 10.1007/PL00000914

[89] Durr UH, Sudheendra US, Ramamoorthy A. LL-37, the only human member of the cathelicidin family of antimicrobial peptides. Biochimica et Biophysica Acta. 2006;**1758**(9):1408-1425. DOI: 10.1016/j.bbamem.2006.03.030

[90] Murakami M, Tonouchi H, Takahashi R, Kitazawa H, Kawai Y, Negishi H, et al. Structural analysis of a new anti-hypertensive peptide (beta-lactosin B) isolated from a commercial whey product. Journal of Dairy Science. 2004;**87**:1967-1974

[91] Murakami M, Dorschner RA, Stern LJ, Lin KH, Gallo RL. Expression and secretion of cathelicidin antimicrobial peptides in murine mammary glands and human milk. Pediatric Research. 2005;**57**:10-15. DOI: 10.1203/01.PDR.0000148068.32201.50

[92] Boman HG. Antibacterial peptides: Basic facts and emerging concepts. Journal of Internal Medicine. 2003;**254**: 197-215. DOI: 10.1046/j.1365-2796.2003.01228.x

[93] Dorschner RA, Lin KH, Murakami M, Gallo RL. Neonatal skin in mice and humans expresses increased levels of antimicrobial peptides: Innate immunity during development of the adaptive response. Pediatric Research. 2003;**53**:566-572. DOI: 10.1203/01.PDR.0000057205.64451.B7

[94] Chen X, Niyonsaba F, Ushio H, Okuda D, Nagaoka I, Ikeda S, et al. Synergistic effect of antibacterial agents human beta-defensins, cathelicidin LL-37 and lysozyme against *Staphylococcus aureus* and *Escherichia coli*. Journal of Dermatological Science. 2005;**40**(2): 123-132. DOI: 10.1016/j.jdermsci.2005.03.014

[95] Scheid A, Li N, Jeffers C, Borriello F, Joshi S, Ozonoff A, et al. Antimicrobial peptide LL-37 and recombinant human mannose-binding lectin express distinct age- and pathogen-specific antimicrobial activity in human newborn cord blood in vitro. F1000Research. 2018;**7**:616. DOI: 10.12688/f1000research.14736.1

[96] Yekta MA, Verdonck F, Van Den Broeck W, Goddeeris BM, Cox E, Vanrompay D. Lactoferrin inhibits *E. coli* O157:H7 growth and attachment to intestinal epithelial cells. Veterinární Medicína. 2010;**55**(8):359-368

[97] Gifford JL, Hunter HN, Vogel HJ. Lactoferricin: A lactoferrin-derived peptide with antimicrobial, antiviral, antitumor and immunological properties. Cellular and Molecular Life Sciences. 2005;**62**:2588-2598. DOI: 10.1007/s00018-005-5373-z

[98] Wakabayashi H, Teraguchi S, Tamura Y. Increased Staphylococcus-killing activity of an antimicrobial peptide, lactoferricin B, with minocycline and monoacylglycerol. Bioscience, Biotechnology, and Biochemistry. 2002;**66**:161-2167. DOI: 10.1271/bbb.66.2161

[99] Bruni N, Capucchio MT, Biasibetti E, Pessione E, Cirrincione S, Giraudo L, et al. Antimicrobial activity of lactoferrin-related peptides and applications in human and veterinary medicine. Molecules. 2016;**21**:E752. DOI: 10.3390/molecules21060752

[100] Brouwer CP, Rahman M, Welling MM. Discovery and development of a synthetic peptide derived from lactoferrin for clinical use. Peptides. 2011;**32**:1953-1963. DOI: 10.1016/j.peptides.2011.07.017

[101] Fu Y, Ji C, Chen X, Cui X, Wang X, Feng J, et al. Investigation into the antimicrobial action and mechanism of a novel endogenous peptide β-casein 197 from human milk. AMB Express. 2017; **7**(1):119. DOI: 10.1186/s13568-017-0409-y

[102] Sun Y, Zhou Y, Liu X, Zhang F, Yan L, Chen L, et al. Wang J antimicrobial activity and mechanism of PDC213, an endogenous peptide from human milk. Biochemical and Biophysical Research Communications. 2017;**484**(1):132-137. DOI: 10.1016/j.bbrc.2017.01.059

[103] WHO. Newborns: Reducing mortality. 2018. Retrieved from: http://www.who.int

[104] WHO Fact Sheet. 2019. Available from: https://www.who.int/news-room/fact-sheets/detail/newborns-reducing-mortality

[105] Camacho-Gonzalez A, Spearman PW, Stoll BJ. Neonatal infectious diseases: Evaluation of neonatal sepsis. Pediatric Clinics of North America. 2013;**60**(2):367-389. DOI: 10.1016/j.pcl.2012.12.003

[106] Verani JR, McGee L, Schrag SJ. Prevention of perinatal group B streptococcal disease–revised guidelines from CDC, 2010. MMWR - Recommendations and Reports. 2010; **59**:1-36

[107] Schrag SJ, Zywicki S, Farley MM, Reingold AL, Harrison LH, Lefkowitz LB, et al. Group B streptococcal disease in the era of intrapartum antibiotic prophylaxis. The New England Journal of Medicine. 2000;**342**:15-20. DOI: 10.1056/NEJM200001063420103

[108] Stoll BJ, Hansen NI, Sanchez PJ, Faix RG, Poindexter BB, Van Meurs KP, et al. Early onset neonatal sepsis: The burden of group B Streptococcal and *E. coli* disease continues. Pediatrics. 2011; **127**:817-826. DOI: 10.1542/peds.2010-2217

[109] Tsai CH, Chen YY, Wang KG, Chen CY, Chen CP. Characteristics of early-onset neonatal sepsis caused by *Escherichia coli*. Taiwanese Journal of Obstetrics & Gynecology. 2012;**51**: 26-30. DOI: 10.1016/j.tjog.2012.01.006

[110] Didier C, Streicher MP, Chognot D, Campagni R, Schnebelen A, Messer J, et al. Late-onset neonatal infections: Incidences and pathogens in the era of antenatal antibiotics. European Journal of Pediatrics. 2012;**171**:681-687. DOI: 10.1007/s00431-011-1639-7

[111] Lim WH, Lien R, Huang YC, Chiang MC, Fu RH, Chu SM, et al. Prevalence and pathogen distribution of neonatal sepsis among very-low-birth-weight infants. Pediatrics and Neonatology. 2012;**53**:228-234. DOI: 10.1016/j.pedneo.2012.06.003

[112] Shane AL, Hansen NI, Stoll BJ, Bell EF, Sánchez PJ, Shankaran S, et al. Methicillin-resistant and susceptible *Staphylococcus aureus* bacteremia and meningitis in preterm infants. Pediatrics. 2012;**129**:e914-e922. DOI: 10.1542/peds.2011-0966

[113] Thompson AM, Bizzarro MJ. Necrotizing enterocolitis in newborns: Pathogenesis, prevention and management. Drugs. 2008;**68**(9): 1227-1238. DOI: 10.2165/00003495-200868090-00004

[114] Coggins SA, Wynn JL, Weitkamp JH. Infectious causes of necrotizing enterocolitis. Clinics in Perinatology. 2015;**42**(1):133-154. DOI: 10.1016/j.clp.2014.10.012

[115] Goerens A, Lehnick D, Büttcher M, Daetwyler K, Fontana M, Genet P, et al. Neonatal ventilator associated pneumonia: A quality improvement initiative focusing on antimicrobial stewardship. Frontiers in Pediatrics. 2018;**24**(6):262. DOI: 10.3389/fped.2018.00262

[116] Bradley JS. Considerations unique to pediatrics for clinical trial design in hospital-acquired pneumonia and ventilator-associated pneumonia. Clinical

Infectious Diseases. 2010;**51**(Suppl 1): S136-S143. DOI: 10.1086/653063

[117] Cantey JB, Wozniak PS, Pruszynski JE, Sanchez PJ. Reducing unnecessary antibiotic use in the neonatal intensive care unit (SCOUT): A prospective interrupted time-series study. The Lancet Infectious Diseases. 2016;**16**:1178-1184. DOI: 10.1016/S1473-3099(16)30205-5

[118] Bhutta ZA, Black RE. Global maternal, newborn, and child health—So near and yet so far. The New England Journal of Medicine. 2013;**369**: 2226-2235. DOI: 10.1056/NEJMra1111853

[119] Turin CG, Ochoa TJ. The role of maternal breast milk in preventing infantile diarrhea in the developing world. Current Tropical Medicine Reports. 2014;**1**(2):97-105. DOI: 10.1007/s40475-014-0015-x

[120] Chirico G, Marzollo R, Cortinovis S, Fonte C, Gasparoni A. Anti-infective properties of human milk. Journal of Nutrition. 2008;**138**(9):1801s-1806s. DOI: 10.1093/jn/138.9.1801S

[121] Lamberti LM, Fischer Walker CL, Noiman A, Victora C, Black RE. Breastfeeding and the risk for diarrhea morbidity and mortality. BMC Public Health. 2011;**11**:S15. DOI: 10.1186/1471-2458-11-S3-S15

[122] Li R, Dee D, Li CM, Hoffman HJ, Grummer-Strawn LM. Breastfeeding and risk of infections at 6 years. Pediatrics. 2014;**134**(Suppl 1):S13-S20. DOI: 10.1542/peds.2014-0646D

[123] Chamova R, Pancheva R, Dimitrova T, Bliznakova D. Protective effect of breast milk on urinary tract infection in children aged 0–3 years. Journal of IMAB - Annual Proceeding (Scientific Papers). 2018;**24**(1): 1918-1922. DOI: 10.5272/jimab.2018241.1918

[124] Black RE, Victora CG, Walker SP, Bhutta ZA, Christian P, de Onis M, et al. Maternal and child under nutrition and overweight in low-income and middle-income countries. Lancet. 2013; **382**(9890):427-451. DOI: 10.1016/S0140-6736(13)60937-X

[125] Ashraf RN, Jalil F, Zaman S, Karlberg J, Khan SR, Lindblad BS, et al. Breast feeding and protection against neonatal sepsis in a high risk population. Archives of Disease in Childhood. 1991; **66**(4):488-490. DOI: 10.1136/adc.66.4.488

[126] Cesar JA, Victora CG, Barros FC, Santos IS, Flores JA. Impact of breast feeding on admission for pneumonia during post-neonatal period in Brazil: Nested case-control study. BMJ. 1999; **318**(7194):1316-1320. DOI: 10.1136/bmj.318.7194.1316

[127] Arifeen S, Black RE, Antelman G, Baqui A, Caulfield L, Becker S. Exclusive breastfeeding reduces acute respiratory infection and diarrhea deaths among infants in Dhaka slums. Pediatrics. 2001;**108**(4):E67. DOI: 10.1542/peds.108.4.e67

[128] Bachrach VR, Schwarz E, Bachrach LR. Breastfeeding and the risk of hospitalization for respiratory disease in infancy: A meta-analysis. Archives of Pediatrics & Adolescent Medicine. 2003;**157**(3):237-243. DOI: 10.1001/archpedi.157.3.237

[129] Meinzen-Derr J, Poindexter B, Wrage L, Morrow AL, Stoll B, Donovan EF. Role of human milk in extremely low birth weight infants risk of necrotizing enterocolitis or death. Journal of Perinatology. 2009;**29**(1): 57-62. DOI: 10.1038/jp.2008.117

[130] Thibeau S, Boudreaux C. Exploring the use of mothers' own milk as oral care for mechanically ventilated very low-birth-weight preterm infants. Advances in Neonatal Care. 2013;**13**(3):

190-197. DOI: 10.1097/ANC.0b013e318285f8e2

[131] Ghaemi S, Navaei P, Rahimirad S, Behjati M, Kelishadi R. Evaluation of preventive effects of colostrum against neonatal conjunctivitis: A randomized clinical trial. Journal of Education Health Promotion. 2014;**23**(3):63. DOI: 10.4103/2277-9531.134776

[132] Herrmann K, Carroll K. An exclusively human milk diet reduces necrotizing enterocolitis. Breastfeeding Medicine. 2014;**9**(4):184-190. DOI: 10.1089/bfm.2013.0121

[133] Miller J, Tonkin E, Damarell RA, McPhee AJ, Suganuma M, Suganuma H, et al. A systematic review and meta-analysis of human milk feeding and morbidity in very low birth weight infants. Nutrients. 2018;**10**(6):707. DOI: 10.3390/nu10060707

[134] Nelson A, Hultenby K, Hell E, Riedel HM, Brismar H, Flock JI, et al. Staphylococcus epidermidis isolated from newborn infants express pilus-like structures and are inhibited by the cathelicidin-derived antimicrobial peptide LL37. Pediatric Research. 2009; **66**:174-178. DOI: 10.1203/PDR.0b013e3181a9d80c

[135] Starner TD, Agerberth B, Gudmundsson GH, McCray PB. Expression and activity of beta-defensins and LL-37 in the developing human lung. Journal of Immunology. 2005;**174**:1608-1615. DOI: 10.4049/jimmunol.174.3.1608

[136] Jenke ACW, Zilbauer M, Postberg J, Wirth S. Human β-defensin 2 expression in ELBW infants with severe necrotizing enterocolitis. Pediatric Research. 2012;**72**:513-520. DOI: 10.1038/pr.2012.110

[137] Salzman NH, Underwood MA, Bevins CL. Paneth cells, defensins, and the commensal microbiota: A hypothesis on intimate interplay at the intestinal mucosa. Seminars in Immunology. 2007;**19**:70-83. DOI: 10.1016/j.smim.2007.04.002

[138] Tecle T, Tripathi S, Hartshorn KL. Review: Defensins and cathelicidins in lung immunity. Innate Immunity. 2010; **16**:151-159. DOI: 10.1177/1753425910365734

[139] Routsias JG, Karagounis P, Parvulesku G, Legakis NJ, Tsakris A. In vitro bactericidal activity of human beta-defensin 2 against nosocomial strains. Peptides. 2010;**31**:1654-1660. DOI: 10.1016/j.peptides.2010.06.010

[140] Guaraldi F, Salvatori G. Effect of breast and formula feeding on gut microbiota shaping in newborns. Frontiers in Cellular and Infection Microbiology. 2012;**2**:94. DOI: 10.3389/fcimb.2012.00094

[141] Gila-Diaz A, Arribas SM, Algara A, Martín-Cabrejas MA, López de Pablo ÁL, Saenz de Pipaon M, et al. A review of bioactive factors in human breast milk: A focus on prematurity. Nutrients. 2019;**11**(6):1307. DOI: 10.3390/nu11061307

[142] Zucht HD, Raida M, Adermann K, Magert HJ, Forssmann WG. Casocidin-I: A casein-alpha(s2) derived peptide exhibits antibacterial activity. FEBS Letters. 1995;**372**:185-188. DOI: 10.1016/0014-5793(95)00974-e

[143] Ferranti P, Traisci MV, Picariello G, Nasi A, Boschi V, Siervo M, et al. Casein proteolysis in human milk: Tracing the pattern of casein breakdown and the formation of potential bioactive peptides. The Journal of Dairy Research. 2004;**71**:74-87. DOI: 10.1017/s0022029903006599

[144] Armaforte E, Curran E, Huppertz T, Ryan A, Caboni MF, O'Connor PM, et al. Proteins and proteolysis in pre-term and term human

milk and possible implications for infant formulae. International Dairy Journal. 2010;**20**:715-723. DOI: 10.1016/j.idairyj.2010.03.008

[145] Dallas DC, Smink CJ, Robinson RC, Tian T, Guerrero A, Parker EA, et al. Endogenous human milk peptide release is greater after preterm birth than term birth. The Journal of Nutrition. 2015; **145**:425-433. DOI: 10.3945/jn.114.203646

[146] Ronayne de Ferrer PA, Baroni A, Sambucetti ME, López NE, CerianiCernadas JM. Lactoferrin levels in term and preterm milk. Journal of the American College of Nutrition. 2000;**19**: 370-373. DOI: 10.1080/07315724.2000.10718933

[147] Albenzio M, Santillo A, Stolfi I, Manzoni P, Iliceto A, Rinaldi M, et al. Lactoferrin levels in human milk after preterm and term delivery. American Journal of Perinatology. 2016;**33**(11): 1085-1089. DOI: 10.1055/s-0036-1586105

[148] Schanler RJ, Shulman RJ, Lau C. Feeding strategies for premature infants: Beneficial outcomes of feeding fortified human milk versus preterm formula. Pediatrics. 1999; **103**(6):1150-1157. DOI: 10.1542/peds.103.6.1150

[149] Sisk PM, Lovelady CA, Dillard RG, Gruber KJ, O'Shea TM. Early human milk feeding is associated with a lower risk of necrotizing enterocolitis in very low birth weight infants. Journal of Perinatology. 2007;**27**(7):428-433. DOI: 10.1038/sj.jp.7211758

[150] Trend S, Strunk T, Hibbert J, Kok CH, Zhang G, Doherty DA, et al. Antimicrobial protein and peptide concentrations and activity in human breast milk consumed by preterm infants at risk of late-onset neonatal sepsis. PLoS One. 2015;**10**:e0117038. DOI: 10.1371/journal.pone.0117038

[151] Demmelmair H, Prell C, Timby N, Lonnerdal B. Benefits of lactoferrin, osteopontin and milk fat globule membranes for infants. Nutrients. 2017; **9**:817. DOI: 10.3390/nu9080817

[152] Bertino E, Giuliani F, Baricco M, Di Nicola P, Peila C, Vassia C, et al. Benefits of donor milk in the feeding of preterm infants. Early Human Development. 2013;**89**(Suppl 2):S3-S6. DOI: 10.1016/j.earlhumdev.2013.07.008

[153] Underwood MA. Human milk for the premature infant. Pediatric Clinics of North America. 2013;**60**(1):189-207. DOI: 10.1016/j.pcl.2012.09.008

[154] Agostoni C, Buonocore G, Carnielli VP, De Curtis M, Darmaun D, Decsi T, et al. Enteral nutrient supply for preterm infants: Commentary from the European Society of Paediatric Gastroenterology, Hepatology and Nutrition Committee on Nutrition. Journal of Pediatric Gastroenterology and Nutrition. 2010;**50**(1):85-91. DOI: 10.1097/MPG.0b013e3181adaee0

[155] King JC Jr, Cummings GE, Guo N, Trivedi L, Readmond BX, Keane V, et al. A double-blind, placebo-controlled, pilot study of bovine lactoferrin supplementation in bottle-fed infants. Journal of Pediatric Gastroenterology and Nutrition. 2007;**44**:245-251. DOI: 10.1097/01.mpg.0000243435.54958.68

[156] Manzoni P, Rinaldi M, Cattani S, Pugni L, Romeo MG, Messner H, et al. Bovine lactoferrin supplementation for prevention of late-onset sepsis in very low-birth-weight neonates: A randomized trial. Journal of the American Medical Association. 2009; **302**:1421-1428. DOI: 10.1001/jama.2009.1403

[157] Arslanoglu S, Boquien CY, King C, Lamireau D, Tonetto P, Barnett D, et al. Fortification of human milk for preterm infants: Update and recommendations of the European Milk Bank Association

(EMBA) Working Group on Human Milk Fortification. Frontiers in Pediatrics. 2019; **7**:76. DOI: 10.3389/fped.2019.00076

[158] Bizzarro MJ, Gallagher PG. Antibiotic-resistant organisms in the neonatal intensive care unit. Seminars in Perinatology. 2007;**31**(1):26-32. DOI: 10.1053/j.semperi.2007.01.004

[159] Borchardt SM, DeBusscher JH, Tallman PA, Manning SD, Marrs CF, Kurzynski TA, et al. Frequency of antimicrobial resistance among invasive and colonizing group B streptococcal isolates. BMC Infectious Diseases. 2006; **6**:57. DOI: 10.1186/1471-2334-6-57

[160] Alarcon A, Pena P, Salas S, Sancha M, Omenaca F. Neonatal early onset *Escherichia coli* sepsis: Trends in incidence and antimicrobial resistance in the era of intrapartum antimicrobial prophylaxis. The Pediatric Infectious Disease Journal. 2004;**23**:295-299. DOI: 10.1097/00006454-200404000-00004

[161] Kayange N, Kamugisha E, Mwizamholya DL, Jeremiah S, Mshana SE. Predictors of positive blood culture and deaths among neonates with suspected neonatal sepsis in a tertiary hospital, Mwanza-Tanzania. BMC Pediatrics. 2010;**10**:39. DOI: 10.1186/1471-2431-10-39

[162] Gandra S, Klein EY, Pant S, Malhotra-Kumar S, Laxminarayan R. Faropenem consumption is increasing in India. Clinical Infectious Diseases. 2016; **62**(8):1050-1052. DOI: 10.1093/cid/ciw055

[163] Nuti R, Goud NS, Saraswati AP, Alvala R, Alvala M. Antimicrobial peptides: A promising therapeutic strategy in tackling antimicrobial resistance. Current Medicinal Chemistry. 2017;**24**(38):4303-4314. DOI: 10.2174/0929867324666170815102441

[164] Lei J, Sun L, Huang S, Zhu C, Li P, He J, et al. The antimicrobial peptides and their potential clinical applications. American Journal of Translational Research. 2019;**11**(7):3919-3931

[165] Parnanen K, Karkman A, Hultman J, Lyra C, Bengtsson-Palme J, Larsson DGJ, et al. Maternal gut and breast milk microbiota affect infant gut antibiotic resistome and mobile genetic elements. Nature Communications. 2018;**9**(1):3891. DOI: 10.1038/s41467-018-06393-w

[166] Desbois AP, Lang S, Gemmell CG, Coote PJ. Surface disinfection properties of the combination of an antimicrobial peptide, ranalexin, with an endopeptidase, lysostaphin, against methicillin-resistant *Staphylococcus aureus* (MRSA). Journal of Applied Microbiology. 2010;**108**:723-730. DOI: 10.1111/j.1365-2672. 2009.04472.x

[167] Jindal HM, Le C-F, MohdYusof MY, Velayuthan RD, Lee VS, Zain SM, et al. Antimicrobial activity of novel synthetic peptides derived from indolicidin and ranalexin against *Streptococcus pneumoniae*. PLoS One. 2015;**10**:e0128532. DOI: 10.1371/journal.pone.0128532

[168] Dosler S, Mataraci E. In vitro pharmacokinetics of antimicrobial cationic peptides alone and in combination with antibiotics against methicillin resistant *Staphylococcus aureus* biofilms. Peptides. 2013;**49**:53-58. DOI: 10.1016/j. peptides.2013.08.008

[169] Shurko JF, Galega RS, Li C, Lee GC. Evaluation of LL-37 antimicrobial peptide derivatives alone and in combination with vancomycin against *S. aureus*. Journal of Antibiotics (Tokyo). 2018;**71**(11):971-974. DOI: 10.1038/s41429-018-0090-7

[170] Le C-F, Yusof MYM, Hassan MAA, Lee VS, Isa DM, Sekaran SD. In vivo efficacy and molecular docking of designed peptide that exhibits potent anti-pneumococcal activity and

synergizes in combination with penicillin. Scientific Reports. 2015;**5**: 11886. DOI: 10.1038/srep11886

[171] Hou M, Zhang N, Yang J, Meng X, Yang R, Li J, et al. Antimicrobial peptide LL-37 and IDR-1 ameliorate MRSA pneumonia in vivo. Cellular Physiology and Biochemistry. 2013;**32**(3):614-623. DOI: 10.1159/000354465

[172] Zaiou M, Nizet V, Gallo RL. Antimicrobial and protease inhibitory functions of the human cathelicidin (hCAP18/LL-37) prosequence. The Journal of Investigative Dermatology. 2003;**120**:810-816. DOI: 10.1046/j.1523-1747.2003.12132.x

[173] Aguila A, Herrera AG, Morrison D, Cosgrove B, Perojo A, Montesinos I, et al. Bacteriostatic activity of human lactoferrin against *Staphylococcus aureus* is a function of its iron-binding properties and is not influenced by antibiotic resistance. FEMS Immunology and Medical Microbiology. 2001;**31**:145-152. DOI: 10.1111/j.1574-695X.2001.tb00511.x

[174] Bjorn C, Mahlapuu M, Mattsby-Baltzer I, Hakansson J. Anti-infective efficacy of the lactoferrin-derived antimicrobial peptide HLR1r. Peptides. 2016;**81**:21-28. DOI: 10.1016/j.peptides.2016.04.005

[175] Hwang SA, Kruzel ML, Actor JK. Immunomodulatory effects of recombinant lactoferrin during MRSA infection. International Immunopharmacology. 2014;**20**(1): 157-163. DOI: 10.1016/j.intimp.2014.02.029

[176] Marks LR, Clementi EA, Hakansson AP. The human milk protein-lipid complex HAMLET sensitizes bacterial pathogens to traditional antimicrobial agents. PLoS One. 2012;7(8):e43514. DOI: 10.1371/journal.pone.0043514

[177] Alamiri F, Riesbeck K, Hakansson AP. HAMLET, a protein complex from human milk has bactericidal activity and enhances the activity of antibiotics against pathogenic *Streptococci*. Antimicrobial Agents and Chemotherapy. 2019;**63**:e01193-19. DOI: 10.1128/AAC.01193-19

[178] Marks LR, Clementi EA, Hakansson AP. Sensitization of *Staphylococcus aureus* to methicillin and other antibiotics in vitro and in vivo in the presence of HAMLET. PLoS One. 2013;**8**(5):e63158. DOI: 10.1371/journal.pone.0063158

[179] Sherman MP. Lactoferrin and necrotizing enterocolitis. Clinics in Perinatology. 2013;**240**:79-91. DOI: 10.1016/j.clp.2012.12.006

[180] Guntupalli K, Dean N, Morris PE, Bandi V, Margolis B, Rivers E, et al. A phase 2 randomized, double-blind, placebo-controlled study of the safety and efficacy of talactoferrin in patients with severe sepsis. Critical Care Medicine. 2013;**41**:706-716. DOI: 10.1097/CCM.0b013e3182741551

[181] Velden WJ, van Iersel TM, Blijlevens NM, Donnelly JP. Safety and tolerability of the antimicrobial peptide human lactoferrin 1-11 (hLF1-11). BMC Medicine. 2009;7:-44. DOI: 10.1186/1741-7015-7-44

[182] Ward PP, Piddington CS, Cunningham GA, Zhou X, Wyatt RD, Conneely OM. A system for production of commercial quantities of human lactoferrin: A broad spectrum natural antibiotic. Biotechnology (NY). 1995; **13**(5):498-503. DOI: 10.1038/nbt0595-498

[183] Monzani PS, Adona PR, Ohashi OM, Meirelles FV, Wheeler MB. Transgenic bovine as bioreactors: Challenges and perspectives. Bioengineered. 2016;7:123-131. DOI: 10.1080/21655979.2016.1171429

[184] Shepelev MV, Kalinichenko SV, Deykin AV, Korobko IV. Production of recombinant proteins in the milk of transgenic animals: Current state and prospects. Acta Naturae. 2018;**10**(3): 40-47

Chapter 7

Breastfeeding and Gut Microbiota

Bita Najafian and Mohammad Hossein Khosravi

Abstract

Human breast milk (HBM) not only is a source of nutrition for infants but also contains a variety of biologically active components and bacterial species. These molecules and bacteria guide both intestinal microbiota and infantile immune system. Recently published studies have found several vital roles for gut microbiota including effects on the individual's personality, decreased predisposition to the diseases, and a variety of other health-related consequences such as possible therapeutic effects or preventing role. In this chapter the components of human breast milk and its effect on shaping the human gut microbiota have been reviewed.

Keywords: breastfeeding, gut microbiota, breast milk, microbiome

1. Introduction

Today, there is no doubt that human breast milk is the most beneficial source of nutrition for infants which is the result of several years of research and evaluation. Beside known nutrients such as proteins and carbohydrates, human breast milk contains a wide range of biologically active components and microbiota [1]. Previous researches have shown that mother's intestinal microbiome is transferred to her infant through breast milk. This relationship between mother and infant plays the key role in forming a healthy intestinal microbiome which is responsible for protecting against diarrheal and respiratory illnesses as well as asthma, obesity, diabetes, atopy, and other inflammatory diseases such as inflammatory bowel diseases (IBD) [2, 3]. The presence of bacteria in human breast milk not only improves the infantile health but also promotes mother's health by a variety of mechanisms such as preventing mastitis [4]. Human milk oligosaccharides (HMOs) have the main role in developing the intestinal microbiota [1]. Their synthesis is determined by maternal genotype.

Transferring immunity from mother to infant is started from the intrauterine life and is continued by breastfeeding. Breast milk includes antibodies and immunities targeting the mother's gut and airway microbes with which her infant is likely to encounter during the very first months of birth [5]. Recently conducted researches have revealed that breast milk directly modulates the development of immune system in breastfed infants as well as provides passive protection [6].

Colostrum is the most enriched part of the breast milk of immune factors which provides an appropriate immune response when the infant is at risk of exposure to new microbes [7]. Hormones, cytokines, growth factors, chemokines, and immunoglobulins are among the bioactive factors that are transferred to infant via breastfeeding [7, 8]. In this chapter a comprehensive review has been done on the role of breastfeeding and breast milk ingredients in forming infant's intestinal microbiota.

IntechOpen

2. Microbial components of breast milk

Before year 2000, human breast milk (HBM) was considered to be sterile. Martin et al. mentioned the presence of commensal and probiotic bacteria in HBM [9]. *Lactobacillus fermentum* and *Lactobacillus gasseri* were more commonly found in breast milk samples using culture-dependent techniques [10]. Today, lactic acid bacterial strains with proven probiotic activities are referred to as probiotics [11]. Every milliliter of breast milk contains about 1000 colony-forming units of various bacterial species [12, 13]. An estimation reveals that infants receive about 800,000 bacteria from breast milk each day [14]. At birth and during delivery, infants receive a notable dose of microbes through different mechanisms such as vaginal flora which is followed by the first breastfeeding [15]. So, breast milk is the second important source of microbiota seeding in the infant's intestines [16, 17]. This has been proven by several previous epidemiologic studies in which the researchers have reported fundamental differences in gut microbiota between breastfed and formula-fed infants [18, 19]. Previous conducted researches have revealed that infantile stool and breast milk have some microbial strains, such as *Enterococcus*, *Staphylococcus*, *Bifidobacterium*, and *Lactobacillus*, in common [20, 21]. It also has been reported that more daily breastfeeding is attributed to more similarity between mother's milk and infant stool microbiome [17].

Newly developed methods, such as next generation sequencing, have augmented our knowledge regarding microbial composition of human breast milk. *Staphylococcus* and *Streptococcus* have been reported to be the most common microbiota families in the human's breast milk. Other families including *Bifidobacterium*, *Lactobacillus*, and *Enterobacteriaceae* family members are placed in the following ranks [22, 23]. Colostrum contains a more various number of bacterial species than do transitional and mature milk.

So far, we have no idea where the mother's milk microbiota exactly comes from; however a number of theories have come up. The first one considers that retrograde flow of breast milk from the infant's mouth to the areola and commensal skin area contaminates the milk with maternal skin flora; however, the presence of anaerobic species does not justify the commensal contamination [24–26]. On the other hand, *Streptococcus* which is abundant in salivary flora is also common in human breast milk microbiome, supporting the retrograde flow theory [27]. The theory of retrograde flow was first mentioned by Ramsay and colleagues where they used ultrasound technology to study the huge transmission of breast milk from the infant's mouth to the mammary gland ducts [25]. Another theory holds this belief that breast milk microbiota are originated from mother's intestinal flora, where they migrate via blood and lymphatic circulation to the mammary glands [27, 28]. Studying pregnant and lactating mice revealed that both aerobic and anaerobic organisms are translocated from gut to the mesenteric lymph nodes and mammary glands, subsequently [28]. In addition, another research team found that there are similar bacterial signatures in breast milk, lymph nodes, and dendritic cells (DC) of lactating mice [29]. Hormonal changes in late pregnancy and increased permeability of the intestinal endothelium are considered to have a supporting role for translocation of intestinal bacteria to mammary glands [27]. Hence, the origin of breast milk microbiota should be more investigated.

A variety of maternal factors have effects on the diversity of mother's milk microbiota. Previously published studies have reported that mothers with vaginal delivery have more various microbial species in their breast milk than that of those who deliver by cesarean section [30, 31]. Also, it has been reported that there is no remarkable difference for milk bacterial concentration between different genders or race groups as well as geographical regions [32, 33]. Various types of breast milk have different bacterial concentrations as the colostrum has lower concentrations than do transitional and mature milk. Results from comparative clinical studies have revealed that breast milk bacterial composition is affected by maternal health condition such as obesity, human immunodeficiency virus (HIV), and celiac disease [34, 35]. Also, it is expectable that maternal chemotherapy and antibiotic use decrease the microbial diversity in mother's milk [36, 37].

3. Mammary gland microbiome

Recently, many efforts have been made to determine the mammary gland bacteriome in different ways [38, 39]. Biopsies from different sites of the breast have approved the viability of bacteria by culture. Human breast tissue bacteriome was shown to be similar to those of the human breast milk where the *Proteobacteria* is the main phylum [40]. Also, nipple aspirate fluid (NAF) has been recently used to determine the breast ductal bacteriome. NAF, which is secreted regularly by breast duct endothelial cells, can be easily collected using a syringe connected to the suction cup applied with a negative pressure [41, 42].

4. Infant gut and what breast milk microbiota has to do

4.1 HBM microbiome as anti-infective

It is believed that breast milk microbiota reduces the incidence of bacterial infections through a variety of mechanisms in breastfed infants. Commensal bacteria modulate growth and replication of pathogen bacteria through their antimicrobial power or as a result of competitive exclusion; as the *Escherichia coli*, *Shigella*, or *Salmonella* strains are inhibited by lactobacilli isolated from human breast milk [43, 44]. In a randomized clinical trial, researchers prescribed breast milk lactobacilli to infants between 6 and 12 months of age which reduced the total incidence of infections [45]. There are a variety of studies which have assessed the antimicrobial activity of the intestine; however; more studies should be conducted for assessing antimicrobial specificities of human breast milk.

4.2 Immunomodulatory role

Animal studies have shown an important role for gut microbiota in increasing and modulating immune functions [46–48]. Lymphoid tissue development was shown to be altered in organs such as the spleen, lymph nodes, and thymus when there is a reduced number of microbiota in the animal intestines. The intestines without any germs have shown reduced numbers of IgA-producing cells, lamina propria CD4+ cells, and hypoplastic Peyer's patches [49]. Production of Th1 cytokines including Il-2, Il-12, and TNF-alpha by macrophages has been shown to be augmented by breast milk lactobacillus strains. Recently conducted studies have shown an improved immunologic and better Th1 response in breastfed infants that that of those fed by formula [50]. *Lactobacillus fermentum* and *Lactobacillus salivarius* have been reported as potent activators of natural killer cells and both innate and acquired immunity as a result of in vitro studies [51]. In addition, human milk metagenome has been shown to contain immunomodulatory DNA motifs which may help modulate exaggerated inflammatory responses to bacterial infection [52]. Most of these regulatory effects were not found in non-milk-derived probiotic bacteria [51].

4.3 Anti-allergic role

A protective association has been discovered between human breast milk lactic acid bacteria and allergies. The main etiology of allergy has been described as the disturbance in regulation of immune system [53]. Previously published animal studies have revealed that probiotic bacteria originated from human breast milk, such as *Lactobacillus gasseri* and *Lactobacillus coryniformis*, have a modulatory role for immune response in cow milk protein sensitivity [54]. However, a conducted randomized clinical trial has shown that prescribing probiotics in the first 6 months of life does not reduce the risk of atopic eczema [55]. Other similar studies have reported that prescribing specific *Lactobacillus* and *Bifidobacterium* species to mothers has led to a reduced incidence of infant eczema in the first 2 years of life [56, 57]. This anti-allergy property of probiotics has been attributed to the downregulation in the production of Th2 cytokines by the hygiene hypothesis [54]. Another clinical study has reported that infants who have more *Klebsiella* species, as the dominant bacteria in their gut, have a higher chance for involving with Atopia, whereas the presence of *Viridans streptococci* in the gut microbiome has the contrary role [58].

4.4 Antitumor properties

However not many studies have been conducted for assessing antitumor properties of the gut microbiome; there are some points in the literature [59]. *Enterococcus faecalis* and *Staphylococcus hominis*, which are isolated from human breast milk, have shown some antitumor properties against a breast cancer cell line [60]. Another similar study has reported that a subspecies of *Lactococcus lactis* has shown therapeutic effect against colon cancer [61].

5. Conclusion

In this chapter we went through the definition and application of human breast milk microbiome and its role on building infant gut microbiome as well as infant's health and disease. Also mentioned is that this gut microbiome may play important roles as anti-infective, immunomodulatory, and anticancer properties. As the importance of breast milk microbiome is getting more notices, further studies should be conducted to assess it more and provide some ways for enriching mother's milk microbiome with beneficial bacteria.

Author details

Bita Najafian[1]* and Mohammad Hossein Khosravi[2]

1 Faculty of Medicine, Department of Pediatrics, Baqiyatallah University of Medical Sciences, Tehran, Iran

2 International Otorhinolaryngology Research Association (IORA), Universal Scientific Education and Research Network (USERN), Tehran, Iran

*Address all correspondence to: dr.najafian@yahoo.com

References

[1] Le Doare K, Holder B, Bassett A, Pannaraj PS. Mother's milk: A purposeful contribution to the development of the infant microbiota and immunity. Frontiers in Immunology. 2018;**9**:361

[2] Xu L, Lochhead P, Ko Y, Claggett B, Leong RW, Ananthakrishnan AN. Systematic review with meta-analysis: Breastfeeding and the risk of Crohn's disease and ulcerative colitis. Alimentary Pharmacology & Therapeutics. 2017;**46**(9):780-789

[3] Azad MB, Vehling L, Lu Z, Dai D, Subbarao P, Becker AB, et al. Breastfeeding, maternal asthma and wheezing in the first year of life: A longitudinal birth cohort study. European Respiratory Journal. 2017;**49**(5):1602019

[4] Jiménez E, de Andrés J, Manrique M, Pareja-Tobes P, Tobes R, Martínez-Blanch JF, et al. Metagenomic analysis of milk of healthy and mastitis-suffering women. Journal of Human Lactation. 2015;**31**(3):406-415

[5] Brandtzaeg P. The mucosal immune system and its integration with the mammary glands. The Journal of Pediatrics. 2010;**156**(2):S8-S15

[6] Mueller NT, Bakacs E, Combellick J, Grigoryan Z, Dominguez-Bello MG. The infant microbiome development: Mom matters. Trends in Molecular Medicine. 2015;**21**(2):109-117

[7] Ballard O, Morrow AL. Human milk composition: Nutrients and bioactive factors. Pediatric Clinics. 2013;**60**(1):49-74

[8] Andreas NJ, Kampmann B, Le-Doare KM. Human breast milk: A review on its composition and bioactivity. Early Human Development. 2015;**91**(11):629-635

[9] Civardi E, Garofoli F, Tzialla C, Paolillo P, Bollani L, Stronati M. Microorganisms in human milk: Lights and shadows. The Journal of Maternal-Fetal & Neonatal Medicine. 2013;**26**(sup2):30-34

[10] Martín R, Langa S, Reviriego C, Jimínez E, Marín ML, Xaus J, et al. Human milk is a source of lactic acid bacteria for the infant gut. The Journal of Pediatrics. 2003;**143**(6):754-758

[11] Mohania D, Nagpal R, Kumar M, Bhardwaj A, Yadav M, Jain S, et al. Molecular approaches for identification and characterization of lactic acid bacteria. Journal of Digestive Diseases. 2008;**9**(4):190-198

[12] Cabrera-Rubio R, Collado MC, Laitinen K, Salminen S, Isolauri E, Mira A. The human milk microbiome changes over lactation and is shaped by maternal weight and mode of delivery. The American Journal of Clinical Nutrition. 2012;**96**(3):544-551

[13] Jeurink P, Van Bergenhenegouwen J, Jiménez E, Knippels L, Fernández L, Garssen J, et al. Human milk: A source of more life than we imagine. Beneficial Microbes. 2013;**4**(1):17-30

[14] Heikkilä MP, Saris P. Inhibition of *Staphylococcus aureus* by the commensal bacteria of human milk. Journal of Applied Microbiology. 2003;**95**(3):471-478

[15] Dominguez-Bello MG, Costello EK, Contreras M, Magris M, Hidalgo G, Fierer N, et al. Delivery mode shapes the acquisition and structure of the initial microbiota across multiple body habitats in newborns. Proceedings of the National Academy of Sciences. 2010;**107**(26):11971-11975

[16] Gritz EC, Bhandari V. The human neonatal gut microbiome: A brief review. Frontiers in Pediatrics. 2015;**3**:17

[17] Pannaraj PS, Li F, Cerini C, Bender JM, Yang S, Rollie A, et al. Association between breast milk bacterial communities and establishment and development of the infant gut microbiome. JAMA Pediatrics. 2017;**171**(7):647-654

[18] Azad MB, Konya T, Maughan H, Guttman DS, Field CJ, Chari RS, et al. Gut microbiota of healthy Canadian infants: Profiles by mode of delivery and infant diet at 4 months. CMAJ. 2013;**185**(5):385-394

[19] Gomez-Llorente C, Plaza-Diaz J, Aguilera M, Muñoz-Quezada S, Bermudez-Brito M, Peso-Echarri P, et al. Three main factors define changes in fecal microbiota associated with feeding modality in infants. Journal of Pediatric Gastroenterology and Nutrition. 2013;**57**(4):461-466

[20] Martín V, Maldonado-Barragán A, Moles L, Rodriguez-Baños M, Campo RD, Fernández L, et al. Sharing of bacterial strains between breast milk and infant feces. Journal of Human Lactation. 2012;**28**(1):36-44

[21] Benito D, Lozano C, Jiménez E, Albújar M, Gómez A, Rodríguez JM, et al. Characterization of *Staphylococcus aureus* strains isolated from faeces of healthy neonates and potential mother-to-infant microbial transmission through breastfeeding. FEMS Microbiology Ecology. 2015;**91**(3):fiv007

[22] Hunt KM, Foster JA, Forney LJ, Schütte UM, Beck DL, Abdo Z, et al. Characterization of the diversity and temporal stability of bacterial communities in human milk. PLoS One. 2011;**6**(6)

[23] Fitzstevens JL, Smith KC, Hagadorn JI, Caimano MJ, Matson AP, Brownell EA. Systematic review of the human milk microbiota. Nutrition in Clinical Practice. 2017;**32**(3):354-364

[24] Urbaniak C, Gloor GB, Brackstone M, Scott L, Tangney M, Reid G. The microbiota of breast tissue and its association with breast cancer. Applied and Environmental Microbiology. 2016;**82**(16):5039-5048

[25] Ramsay DT, Kent JC, Owens RA, Hartmann PE. Ultrasound imaging of milk ejection in the breast of lactating women. Pediatrics. 2004;**113**(2):361-367

[26] Biagi E, Quercia S, Aceti A, Beghetti I, Rampelli S, Turroni S, et al. The bacterial ecosystem of mother's milk and infant's mouth and gut. Frontiers in Microbiology. 2017;**8**:1214

[27] Rodríguez JM. The origin of human milk bacteria: Is there a bacterial entero-mammary pathway during late pregnancy and lactation? Advances in Nutrition. 2014;**5**(6):779-784

[28] Perez PF, Doré J, Leclerc M, Levenez F, Benyacoub J, Serrant P, et al. Bacterial imprinting of the neonatal immune system: Lessons from maternal cells? Pediatrics. 2007;**119**(3):e724-ee32

[29] Zhou X, Voigt A, Paveglio S, Weinstock G, Matson A, Davidovics Z. Similar bacterial signatures in intestinal tissues, milk, and dendritic cells of lactating mice suggest a possible entero-mammary pathway. Gastroenterology. 2017;**152**(5):S172

[30] Cabrera-Rubio R, Mira-Pascual L, Mira A, Collado M. Impact of mode of delivery on the milk microbiota composition of healthy women. Journal of Developmental Origins of Health and Disease. 2016;**7**(1):54-60

[31] Khodayar-Pardo P, Mira-Pascual L, Collado M, Martínez-Costa C. Impact of lactation stage, gestational age and mode of delivery on breast milk

microbiota. Journal of Perinatology. 2014;**34**(8):599-605

[32] Urbaniak C, Angelini M, Gloor GB, Reid G. Human milk microbiota profiles in relation to birthing method, gestation and infant gender. Microbiome. 2016;**4**(1):1

[33] Kumar H, du Toit E, Kulkarni A, Aakko J, Linderborg KM, Zhang Y, et al. Distinct patterns in human milk microbiota and fatty acid profiles across specific geographic locations. Frontiers in Microbiology. 2016;**7**:1619

[34] Olivares M, Albrecht S, De Palma G, Ferrer MD, Castillejo G, Schols HA, et al. Human milk composition differs in healthy mothers and mothers with celiac disease. European Journal of Nutrition. 2015;**54**(1):119-128

[35] González R, Mandomando I, Fumadó V, Sacoor C, Macete E, Alonso PL, et al. Breast milk and gut microbiota in African mothers and infants from an area of high HIV prevalence. PLoS One. 2013;**8**(11)

[36] Soto A, Martín V, Jiménez E, Mader I, Rodríguez JM, Fernández L. Lactobacilli and bifidobacteria in human breast milk: Influence of antibiotherapy and other host and clinical factors. Journal of Pediatric Gastroenterology and Nutrition. 2014;**59**(1):78

[37] Urbaniak C, McMillan A, Angelini M, Gloor GB, Sumarah M, Burton JP, et al. Effect of chemotherapy on the microbiota and metabolome of human milk, a case report. Microbiome. 2014;**2**(1):24

[38] Urbaniak C, Cummins J, Brackstone M, Macklaim JM, Gloor GB, Baban CK, et al. Microbiota of human breast tissue. Applied and Environmental Microbiology. 2014;**80**(10):3007-3014

[39] Hieken TJ, Chen J, Hoskin TL, Walther-Antonio M, Johnson S, Ramaker S, et al. The microbiome of aseptically collected human breast tissue in benign and malignant disease. Scientific Reports. 2016;**6**:30751

[40] Murphy K, Curley D, O'Callaghan TF, O'Shea C-A, Dempsey EM, O'Toole PW, et al. The composition of human milk and infant faecal microbiota over the first three months of life: A pilot study. Scientific Reports. 2017;**7**(1):1-10

[41] Chan AA, Bashir M, Rivas MN, Duvall K, Sieling PA, Pieber TR, et al. Characterization of the microbiome of nipple aspirate fluid of breast cancer survivors. Scientific Reports. 2016;**6**(1):1-11

[42] Petrakis NL. Nipple aspirate fluid in epidemiologic studies of breast disease. Epidemiologic Reviews. 1993;**15**(1):188-195

[43] Jara S, Sánchez M, Vera R, Cofré J, Castro E. The inhibitory activity of Lactobacillus spp. isolated from breast milk on gastrointestinal pathogenic bacteria of nosocomial origin. Anaerobe. 2011;**17**(6):474-477

[44] Lyons A, O'mahony D, O'brien F, MacSharry J, Sheil B, Ceddia M, et al. Bacterial strain-specific induction of Foxp3+ T regulatory cells is protective in murine allergy models. Clinical and Experimental Allergy. 2010;**40**(5):811-819

[45] Maldonado J, Cañabate F, Sempere L, Vela F, Sánchez AR, Narbona E, et al. Human milk probiotic *Lactobacillus fermentum* CECT5716 reduces the incidence of gastrointestinal and upper respiratory tract infections in infants. Journal of Pediatric Gastroenterology and Nutrition. 2012;**54**(1):55-61

[46] Arrieta M-C, Stiemsma LT, Amenyogbe N, Brown EM, Finlay B. The intestinal microbiome in early life:

Health and disease. Frontiers in Immunology. 2014;**5**:427

[47] Gensollen T, Iyer SS, Kasper DL, Blumberg RS. How colonization by microbiota in early life shapes the immune system. Science. 2016;**352**(6285):539-544

[48] Walker WA, Iyengar RS. Breast milk, microbiota, and intestinal immune homeostasis. Pediatric Research. 2015;**77**(1-2):220-228

[49] Macpherson AJ, Harris NL. Interactions between commensal intestinal bacteria and the immune system. Nature Reviews. Immunology. 2004;**4**(6):478-485

[50] Pabst H, Spady D, Pilarski L, Carson M, Beeler J, Krezolek M. Differential modulation of the immune response by breast-or formula-feeding of infants. Acta Paediatrica. 1997;**86**(12):1291-1297

[51] Perez-Cano FJ, Dong H, Yaqoob P. In vitro immunomodulatory activity of *Lactobacillus fermentum* CECT5716 and *Lactobacillus salivarius* CECT5713: Two probiotic strains isolated from human breast milk. Immunobiology. 2010;**215**(12):996-1004

[52] Ward TL, Hosid S, Ioshikhes I, Altosaar I. Human milk metagenome: A functional capacity analysis. BMC Microbiology. 2013;**13**(1):116

[53] Prokopakis E, Vardouniotis A, Kawauchi H, Scadding G, Georgalas C, Hellings P, et al. The pathophysiology of the hygiene hypothesis. International Journal of Pediatric Otorhinolaryngology. 2013;**77**(7): 1065-1071

[54] Lara-Villoslada F, Olivares M, Sierra S, Rodríguez JM, Boza J, Xaus J. Beneficial effects of probiotic bacteria isolated from breast milk. British Journal of Nutrition. 2007;**98**(S1):S96-S100

[55] Taylor AL, Dunstan JA, Prescott SL. Probiotic supplementation for the first 6 months of life fails to reduce the risk of atopic dermatitis and increases the risk of allergen sensitization in high-risk children: A randomized controlled trial. Journal of Allergy and Clinical Immunology. 2007;**119**(1):184-191

[56] Abrahamsson TR, Jakobsson T, Böttcher MF, Fredrikson M, Jenmalm MC, Björkstén B, et al. Probiotics in prevention of IgE-associated eczema: A double-blind, randomized, placebo-controlled trial. Journal of Allergy and Clinical Immunology. 2007;**119**(5):1174-1180

[57] Kim JY, Kwon JH, Ahn SH, Lee SI, Han YS, Choi YO, et al. Effect of probiotic mix (*Bifidobacterium bifidum*, *Bifidobacterium lactis*, *Lactobacillus acidophilus*) in the primary prevention of eczema: A double-blind, randomized, placebo-controlled trial. Pediatric Allergy and Immunology. 2010;**21**(2p2):e386-ee93

[58] Kirjavainen PV, Apostolou E, Arvola T, Salminen SJ, Gibson GR, Isolauri E. Characterizing the composition of intestinal microflora as a prospective treatment target in infant allergic disease. FEMS Immunology and Medical Microbiology. 2001;**32**(1):1-7

[59] Ojo-Okunola A, Nicol M, Du Toit E. Human breast milk bacteriome in health and disease. Nutrients. 2018;**10**(11):1643

[60] Hassan Z, Mustafa S, Rahim RA, Isa NM. Anti-breast cancer effects of live, heat-killed and cytoplasmic fractions of *Enterococcus faecalis* and *Staphylococcus hominis* isolated from human breast milk. In Vitro Cellular & Developmental Biology. Animal. 2016;**52**(3):337-348

[61] Kim JY, Woo HJ, Kim Y-S, Kim KH, Lee HJ. Cell cycle dysregulation induced by cytoplasm of *Lactococcus lactis* ssp. lactis in SNUC2A, a colon cancer cell line. Nutrition and Cancer. 2003;**46**(2):197-201

Section 5

Formula Feeding: Thermal Processing Contaminants

Chapter 8

The Evaluation of Childhood Foods and Infant Formula Exposure to Furan, Chloropropanols and Acrylamide Contamination by Food Processing

Burhan Başaran

Abstract

This review attempted to evaluate the exposure of thermal processing contaminants such as furan, chloropropanols and acrylamide from infant formulas. Furan, chloropropanols and acrylamide exist at varying levels in several types of foods that are consumed in daily diet including infant formulas. The consumption of these foods leads to the exposure to the thermal processing contaminants. In this sense, it is apparent that humans face hidden danger through dietary exposure throughout their lives. Infants are considered as the age group that expose to the highest levels of these substances as a result of the fact that they have low body weight and consume infant formulas in their diets as alternative nutrition. The review emphasizes that the infant formulas are not innocent, on the contrary, they can be considered as safety critical for infants considering that infant formulas include furan, chloropropanols and acrylamide. Therefore, this review suggests that in this sense all shareholders' (university, non-governmental organizations, public and private sector) acting in concert with each other is crucially important for the health of individuals and overall society.

Keywords: infant formulas, furan, chloropropanols, 3-MCPD, 2-MCPD, glycidol, acrylamide, exposure

1. Introduction

World Health Organization (WHO) and UNICEF advices that infants need to be exclusively breasted for the first 6 months and breastfeeding should last minimum 2 years. Nevertheless, around the world, the rate of breastfeeding in the first 6 months is still 38% and this percentage has not changed for about 20 years. It is known that breast milk significantly contributes to infants' physical and mental development and acts as a protector for infants against several diseases. Therefore, with the contributions of WHO and UNICEF, breast milk is being promoted in order to increase the rate of breastfeeding to 50% for the first 6 months until 2025 and studies are being carried out with regard to the importance of breast feeding in early periods of infancy [1, 2].

Use of breast feeding as primary nutrition in early periods, namely in the first 6 months, of infancy is highly common around the world (Norway: 95%, Australia: 92%, Canada: 89%, United States: 77%) and the percentage increases gradually year by year. On the contrary, after 6 months is decreasing dramatically [3]. By all means, there are several factors affecting this case. Some of these factors are mothers' becoming a mother young, not having breastfeeding experience, concern of insufficient breast milk, desire to feed their babies with new tastes, active work life, long working hours and perceptions of mothers created by other individuals, mother's and baby's health condition, babies' becoming acquainted with pacifier and feeding bottle [4–6]. Besides these factors, depending on the development of the baby, mothers generally give their babies other nourishments as supplement to breast milk or use them as only source of nutrition for their babies. The top of these nourishments is infant formulas.

There are several firms operating globally in the sector of infant formulas which has become a massive market today. These firms invest in research-development activities, advertising activities and develop marketing strategies in order to gain advantage in the competition [7]. It is easy to find several follow-on milk, follow-on formulas and mixed formulas for the needs of 0–6 months-old and >6 months-old babies, which are formulated either in powder or liquid form and enriched with various ingredients [8]. Infant formulas are often preferred in that they are accessible and easy to prepare; besides, they can be used by others when mother is not available for feeding. On the other hand, it is known that mothers are deeply anxious about the infant formulas although they try to make their best to choose the most appropriate formula for their babies based on their research on written and visual media, advices from others and past experiences [9, 10].

On one hand, it is beyond argument that breast milk is the best choice for babies' nourishment, development and health; on the other hand, it is not always the one and only choice because of various reasons. Therefore, it needs to be ensured that the adverse effects of infant formulas, which are used as supplement to breast milk or used exclusively, on babies' health in the short-, medium- and long-term are eliminated and these formulas not to cause any health problems for babies. In this respect, certain legal regulations are designed for the production and marketing of infant formulas nationally and globally. However, in the literature, although infant formulas carry the risk with respect to furan, acrylamide, chloropropanols and polycyclic aromatic hydrocarbons, which are called thermal processing contaminants and have potential to cause various health problems for humans, this information has not been referred in the legal regulations. Considering that the contaminants in question are included in various foods that are frequently preferred in daily diets, individuals expose to these contaminants starting from very early periods of infancy and this exposure continues throughout their lives. To this end, the current review aims to evaluate the infant formulas with respect to certain thermal processing contaminants.

2. Thermal process contaminants

Besides bringing certain sensorial properties to foods, thermal process is a processing technique that eliminates or decreases the potential hazards originating from foods against consumers' health through making foods microbiologically more reliable. However, under certain conditions thermal processing applications cause certain toxic substances called "thermal processing contaminants" (heterocyclic aromatic amines, 5-hydroxymethylfurfural, polycyclic aromatic hydrocarbons, nitrosamines, furan, acrylamide, and chloropropanols) to emerge [11, 12]. In the last 10 years, a great amount of research has focused on thermal processing contaminants and this topic is still current and important for consumers, health authorities and industries [13].

2.1 Furan

Furan is colorless, highly volatile and flammable compound with a boiling point close to room temperature (≈31°C). It is soluble in most of the organic solvents such as alcohol and acetone. Furan with a molecular formula of C_4H_4O and CAS number of 110-00-9 is a heterocyclic and aromatic compound [14].

Formation of furan in foods is the result of various mechanisms. It has been documented that besides the presence of reducing sugar or amino acids, thermal degradation or Maillard reaction, ascorbic acid, thermal oxidation, oxidized polyunsaturated lipids, serine and cysteine without other sources [15, 16].

In the risk assessment undertaken by U.S. National Institutes of Health (NIH) and Joint FAO/WHO Expert Committee on Food Additives (JECFA) depending on the studies on laboratory animals, furan was reported to be a strong carcinogenic compound that affected several organs [17, 18]. It has been identified as "possibly carcinogen to humans" (Group 2B) by International Agency for Research on Cancer (IARC) [19].

In a study conducted by The US Food and Drug Administration (FDA) in year 2004 with 334 foodstuffs, presence of furan was reported for canned and jarred baby foods, infant formulas, coffees, meats, fish, soups, sauces, vegetables and fruits and several other foodstuffs that underwent thermal processing. Particularly, the study reported that all baby foods included furan [20]. After FD reports, The European Commission Recommendation 2007/196/EC offered a suggestion to the member countries in order for tracking the toxicity, formation, analysis and the exposure of furan [21]. Based on the reports from several countries, JECFA reported the foodstuffs that included the highest furan levels; roasted coffee (powder) (814–4590 μg/kg), instant coffee (powder) (90–783 μg/kg), brewed roasted coffee (34–113 μg/kg), baby food (19–96 μg/kg), soya sauce (16–52 μg/kg), canned fish (6–76 μg/kg) and baked beans (27–581 μg/kg) [22]. According to the reports of European Food Safety Authority (EFSA) and FDA, Crews and Castle classified the foodstuffs in three categories that included furan more than 100 μg/kg; coffee, baby foods, sauces and soups. Moreover, furan was found in 262 of 273 baby foods, 70 of 71 infant foods, 28 of 42 infant formulas. The levels of furan in baby foods, infant foods and infant formulas change between the ranges of 1–112 μg/kg (mean: 28 μg/kg), 1.3–87.3 μg/kg (mean: 27 μg/kg) and 2.5–27 μg/kg (mean: 12 μg/kg), respectively [23]. Several studies reported different levels of furan in baby foods and infant formulas; EFSA 31–32, 0.2–3.2 μg/kg, Liu and Tsai 4.23–124.1, 2.4–28.7 μg/kg [24, 25]. Lambert et al. determined the furan levels of many foods including baby foods and infant formulas (**Table 1**) [26].

In this respect, **Table 2** displays the results of dietary exposure of furan in individuals from diverse group of ages reported by EFSA.

The mean of infants' dietary exposure of furan was reported as 0.99–1.34 μg/kg bw per day by FAO/WHO whereas Health Canada reported this level as 1.76 μg/kg bw per day [17, 28]. Some studies reported the mean of dietary exposure of furan for 4 months, 5–6 months, 7–12 months and 13–36 months old infants as 0.14, 0.60, 0.84 and 0.37 μg/kg bw per day [29] and 0.09, 0.56, 0.80 and 0.33 μg/kg bw per day, respectively [30].

Food group	Mean (μg/kg)
Baby foods	3.3–41
Infant formulae	3.5–5.7
Vegetables	5.9–6.3
Fish	5.3–5.3
Cereal products	44–44
Meat products	7.3–7.5
Milk products	1.4–2.3
Soups	16–16

The data were taken directly from Lambert et al.

Table 1.
The mean level of furan in different food groups [26].

Age group	Mean dietary exposure (μg/kg bw per day)	High dietary exposure (μg/kg bw per day)
Infants	0.14–0.99	0.27–1.82
Toddlers	0.22–0.65	0.05–0.31
Other children	0.19–0.52	0.29–0.86
Adolescents	0.11–0.54	0.20–1.22
Adults	0.03–0.59	0.08–1.29
Elderly	0.12–0.61	0.24–1.27
Very elderly	0.13–0.75	0.27–0.96

The data were taken directly from EFSA Journal.

Table 2.
Dietary exposure of furan [27].

2.2 Chloropropanols

In recent years, the presence of chloropropanols (certain fatty acid esters of 3-monochloro-1,2-propanediol (3-MCPD) and the related substance glycidol, 2-monochloro-1,3-propanediol (2-MCPD), 1,3-dichloro-2-propanol (1,3-DCP) and 2,3-dichloro-1-propanol (2,3-DCP)) in foodstuffs has aroused the attention of researchers [31]. Dichloropropanols are comprised of monoesters whereas monochloropropanediols are comprised of both monoesters and diesters [32]. It has been estimated that depending on thermal processing, lipids, glycerol, triolein and lecithin that are heated with hydrochloric acid are precursors in the formation of chloropropanols in foodstuffs [33, 34]. Chloropropanols and its esters are created from lipids and chlorides in the oil refining process particularly when the deodorization process is realized under high temperatures. Moreover, glycidol can occur through dehalogenation from 3-MCPD [35].

It has not been ascertained that whether chloropropanol is a carcinogenic compound. On the other hand, it is disturbing that some free chloropropanol forms in foodstuffs are potentially toxic. The JECFA reported that 1,3-DCP is a genotoxic carcinogen, however, there is not enough evidence for the toxicologic evaluation of 2-MCPD [36, 37]. In this respect, Lee and Khor found that 3-MCPD and 1,3-DCP have potential genotoxic and carcinogenic characteristics [38]. Similarly, Onami et al. suggested that 3-MCPD carries unignorable risks for human health with regard to its potential hazard [39]. In some other studies 1,3-DCP and 3-MCPD are defined as possible human carcinogens (group 2B) and similarly glycidol is referred as a probable human carcinogen (group 2A) [40–42]. One of the most comprehensive studies on the toxicologic evaluation of chloropropanols revealed that whereas the carcinogenic effect of 1,3-DCP was highly evident, for the reason that the level of its presence in foodstuffs was considerably low, 1,3-DCP did not carry a risk for human health. This comprehensive study emphasized the insufficiency of the research on the level of the presence of 2-MCPD and 2,3-DCP in foodstuffs and the toxicologic evaluation of these substances. However, current evidence suggests that these compounds can be considered within low risk group for human health for the reason that the level of the presence of these compounds in foodstuffs is low [43]. EFSA determined the tolerable daily intake (TDI) for 3-MCPD as 0.8 μg/kg bw per day, whereas JECFA suggested the provisional maximum tolerable daily intake (PMTDI) of 4 μg/kg bw/day [44, 45].

Recent studies revealed that chloropropanols was found in several foodstuffs at different levels particularly in soy sauces, meat and meat products, fish and sea foods, cereals, snacks, bread, biscuits, crisps, chips, baby foods and infant formulas as well [46, 47]. **Table 3** shows the levels of chloropropanols in foodstuffs reported in the comprehensive study by EFSA.

Considering the other studies on infant formulas and chloropropanols, Zelinková et al. identified 3-MCPD as 1.04–2.03 mg/kg, Weißhaar identified glycidol as 2.6–5.3 mg/kg, and Wöhrlin et al. identified 3-MCPD as 0.42 mg/kg and 2-MCPD, 0.19 mg/kg, glycidol 0.36 mg/kg [49–51]. **Table 4** displays the results suggested by EFSA regarding the dietary exposure of chloropropanols for the individuals from different age groups.

EFSA revealed that the food group that contributes 50% and higher levels of 3-MCPD, 2-MCPD and glycidol exposure for infants is infant formulas and follow-on formulas, which are followed by vegetable fats and oils, besides cookies. The levels of 3-MCPD, 2-MCPD and glycidol considering the exposure from only infant formulas were calculated as 2.4, 0.7–1.3, and 1.8–2.1 μg/kg bw per day, respectively [48]. JECFA estimated the average exposure to glycidol equivalents for babies between 0.1 and 3.6 μg/kg bw/day. However, the exposure level of 3-MCPD equivalents can increase to 10 μg/kg bw/day on average for the babies that are fed by infant formulas in the early periods of their lives [45]. Spungen et al. estimated the exposure of 3-MCPD equivalents for 0–1, 2–3 and 5–6 months old babies as 10,

Food groups	3-MCPD μg/kg	2-MCPD μg/kg	Glycidol μg/kg
Vegetable fats and oils	1093 (1090–1095)	414 (400–427)	1268 (1259–1277)
Margarine and similar products	408 (406–409)	159 (152–166)	361 (358–364)
Infant formulas (powder)	108 (108–109)	44 (31–58)	87 (80–94)
Cereal-based products and similar	83 (77–90)	42 (38–47)	51 (50–51)
Fried, baked or roast meat or fish products	30 (26–34)	10 (7–14)	38 (38–39)
Smoked meat or fish products	21 (15–28)	6.2 (0.5–11)	17 (15–19)
Snacks and potato products	130 (123–137)	79 (75–84)	58 (58–59)

*The data were taken directly from EFSA Journal.

Table 3.
The mean level of 3-MCPD, 2-MCPD, glycidol and esters in different food groups [48].

Age group	3-MCPD µg/kg bw per day	2-MCPD µg/kg bw per day	Glycidol µg/kg bw per day
Infants	0.5–1.0	0.2–0.4	0.4–0.8
Toddlers	0.6–1.4	0.3–0.6	0.4–0.9
Other children	0.5–1.5	0.3–0.7	0.3–0.9
Adolescents	0.2–0.7	0.1–0.3	0.2–0.5
Adults	0.2–0.4	0.1–0.2	0.2–0.3
Elderly	0.2–0.4	0.1–0.2	0.1–0.3
Very elderly	0.2–0.5	0.1–0.2	0.1–0.3

The data were taken directly from EFSA Journal.

Table 4.
The mean of the dietary exposure to 3-MCPD, 2-MCPD and Glycidol [48].

8, 7 µg/kg bw per day respectively, whereas the exposure of glycidol and esters were estimated 2 µg/kg bw per day and same for all age groups [52]. Arisseto et al. identified the exposure of 3-MCPD for.

0–5, 6–11 months old babies as 2.49, 1.05 µg/kg bw/day, respectively and the glycidol exposure as 3.65, 1.64 µg/kg bw/day [53].

2.3 Acrylamide

Acrylamide (AA), which was identified for the first time as a chemical compound in 1893 in Germany, is a chemical agent used extensively in such sectors as dams, tunnels, water treatment, paper and textile [54]. The presence of AA in foods for the first time was identified in 2002 by a group of researchers in Sweden [55]. Acrylamide formation in foods is explained through several mechanisms. The most important of all these mechanisms is especially Maillard reaction, which is performed in thermal processing with the presence of asparagines amino acid and reducing sugar [56]. It has been revealed that, apart from this mechanism, acrolein, B-alanine, aspartic acid, pyruvic acid and carnosine cause AA formation through various reactions [57].

In the experimental studies carried out with animals, a positive dose-response relationship between AA and the cancer in multi-organs and tissues was found [58, 59]. In epidemiological studies conducted with humans, it was suggested that AA could seriously affect fetal development [60] and neurological changes [61]. On the other hand, there is not a clear consensus on the relationship between AA and cancer yet. Whereas, some studies reveal that AA increases the risk of contracting ovarian cancer [62], lung cancer [63] and the cancers related to digestive and respiratory systems [64], some other studies determine that AA has no positive relationship with several types of cancer [65–67]. However, IARC classifies AA as a probable human carcinogen (group 2A) [68].

EFSA reported the results of the study that show AA levels in several foodstuffs in 2015 (**Table 5**).

In the other studies on infant formulas, different acrylamide levels were reported; Fohgelberg et al. found 3.5–223 µg/kg and Elias et al. found <LOD (limit of detection)-353 µg/kg [70, 71]. Likewise, **Table 6** displays the results of dietary AA exposure of the individuals from different age groups reported by EFSA.

Mojska et al. calculated the daily dietary intake of acrylamide for 6, 7, 8, 9 and 10–12 months old babies as 17.46, 20.87, 21.65, 29.06 and 38.05 µg/person/day, respectively [72]. Considering the other studies on AA exposure, Health Canada estimated the AA exposure for <1 years and 1–3 years old babies as

Food groups	Mean (μg/kg)
Potato fried products (except potato crisps and snacks)	308 (303–313)
Potato crisps and snacks	389 (388–389)
Soft bread	42 (36–49)
Breakfast cereals	161 (157–164)
Biscuits, crackers, crisp bread and similar	265 (261–269)
Coffee (dry)	522 (521–523)
Coffee substitutes (dry)	1499
Baby foods, other than cereal-based	24 (17–31)
Processed cereal-based baby foods	73 (70–76)
Other products based on potatoes, cereals and cocoa	97 (92–101)

*The data were taken directly from EFSA Journal.

Table 5.
AA the mean levels of several foods (μg/kg) [69].

Age group	Mean dietary exposure (μg/kg bw per day)	High dietary exposure (μg/kg bw per day)
Infants	0.5–1.6	1.4–2.5
Toddlers	0.9–1.9	1.4–3.4
Other children	0.9–1.6	1.4–3.2
Adolescents	0.4–0.9	0.9–2.0
Adults	0.4–0.6	0.8–1.3
Elderly	0.4–0.5	0.7–1.0
Very elderly	0.4–0.5	0.6–1.0

*The data were taken directly from EFSA Journal.

Table 6.
The mean of the dietary AA exposure [69].

0.211, 0.609 μg/kg bw per day, respectively, and Sirot et al. found the AA exposure levels for 1–4, 5–6, 7–12 and 13–36 months-old babies as 0.14, 0.03, 0.40 and 0.07 μg/kg bw per day, respectively [30, 73].

3. Acrylamide, furan and chloropropanol exposure caused by breast milk

It is estimated that babies are exposed to contaminants coming from breast milk from the first seconds of their lives. This exposure varies depending on the impact of many factors such as the age of the mother, dietary habits, living space, and environmental contaminants etc. on the compounds in breast milk. Therefore, breast milk is globally monitored as a biomarker for exposure and sheds light on exposure evaluation studies [74, 75].

The number of studies on the acrylamide level of breast milk is very limited. Sörgel et al. detected acrylamide in milk of mothers consuming foods that contain high levels of acrylamide such as potato chips, French fries etc. They stated that 10 to 50% of acrylamide occurring in pregnant women due to nutrition is transferred to the fetus through blood and it can reach μg/L in breast milk. They state that acrylamide exposure caused by breast milk continues until the end of breastfeeding, and therefore nursing mothers should avoid foods containing acrylamide until uncertainties about acrylamide are eliminated [76]. Fohgelberg et al. stated that traces of acrylamide were detected in all breast milk samples, the acrylamide level was determined as 0.51 μg/kg only in one sample while the acrylamide levels in the other 18 samples were under the limit of quantification (0.5 μg/kg). The mean acrylamide level in breast milk was assumed to be 0.25 μg/kg in the study and the mean acrylamide exposure was estimated as 0.04 μg/kg bw per day (the mean body weight is calculated as 5.5 kg) for infants that are fed only with breast milk during the early breastfeeding period. The results revealed the importance of breastfeeding as a way of preventing the baby from being exposed to acrylamide as the level of acrylamide in breast milk is very low [70].

The source and possible consequences of 3-MCPD in breast milk have not been entirely explored yet. However, it has been stated that dietary habits of mothers are an important factor for presence of 3-MCPD in breast milk [34, 77]. Zelinkova et al. determined the 3-MCPD level between 11 and 76 μg/kg and the mean amount as 35.5 μg/kg in 12 breast milk samples. They determined the 3-MCPD exposure caused by breast milk in babies (breastfed for up to 4 months) as 26,625 μg/day (average daily intake of mother's milk by the baby is about 750 mL) and 8.19 μg/kg bw per day [77]. Jędrkiewicz et al. stated that 2-MCPD and 3-MCPD reached 2.2 mg/kg in breast milk and therefore it was highly difficult for babies to avoid chloropropanols [78].

Polychlorinated dibenzofurans (PCDFs), which are another contaminant in breast milk, have been examined in studies together with polychlorinated biphenyls (PCBs) and polychlorinated dibenzo-p-dioxins (PCDDs). A lot of studies can be found in the literature on this subject compared to acrylamide and chloropropanols. As breast milk is the first and most important way of conveying PCBs and PCDD/Fs to babies, WHO has been conducting global studies on dioxin detection in breast milk since 1987 [79]. Costopoulou et al. reported that the countries with the highest level of PCBs and PCDD/Fs in breast milk are Egypt, the Netherlands, Belgium, Luxemburg, and Italy {respectively, 22.3, 18.27, 16.92, 14.97, 12.66 pg/g [fat WHO-TEQ (toxicity equivalent)]} while the countries with the lowest levels are Fiji, Brazil, the Philippines, Australia, and Bulgaria (respectively 3.34, 3.92, 3.94, 5.57 and 6.14 pg/g fat WHO-TEQ) [80]. WHO has estimated the range of tolerable daily dose as 1–4 pg TEQ/kg bs per day for babies exposed to dioxin contaminants such as PCDD/Fs and PCBs [81]. Focant et al. calculated the average concentration for total TEQ (PCDD/Fs and PCBs) as 17.81 pg/g and the daily intake of PCDD/Fs and PCBs as 62.3 TEQ/kg bw per day [82]. In a study they conducted in China (Guangdong Province), Huang et al. predicted the mean EDI level of PCDD/PCBs resulting from breast milk as 54.3 pg TEQ/kg bw per day [83].

4. Conclusion

The current review evaluated infant formulas that have an important place in the diets of babies, with respect to the thermal processing contaminants; furan, chloropropanols and acrylamide, which have become one of the foci of researchers. When the results of the studies regarding the exposure of these contaminants are evaluated, it is suggested that babies are in the risk group, who are highly exposed to these contaminants because of their low body weight compared to other individuals, besides; there are no alternative foods to infant formulas in their daily diet. In the light of the evidence revealed by the previous studies, the current review proposes that regarding the furan, chloropropanols and acrylamide, infant formulas can be a concern for baby health. Nevertheless, the review further suggests that it is important to decrease the level of thermal processing contaminants or specify certain upper limits and determine these regulations by law for the individual health and the health of the overall society. Furthermore, the current review emphasized that infant formulas are not alternatives to breast milk and educating mothers in this respect is critically important for the health of next generations. One last thing to emphasize is the need to raise the awareness of breastfeeding mothers in avoiding the consumption of foods that have a rich content in terms of the abovementioned contaminants.

Author details

Burhan Başaran
Travel, Tourism and Recretaion Department, Ardeşen Vocational School, Recep Tayyip Erdoğan University, Rize, Turkey

*Address all correspondence to: burhan.basaran@erdogan.edu.tr

References

[1] World Health Organization (WHO). Country Implementation of the International Code of Marketing of Breast-Milk Substitutes: Status Report. 2011. Available from: https://apps.who.int/iris/bitstream/handle/10665/85621/9789241505987_eng.pdf [Accessed: 25 May 2020]

[2] UNICEF. Improving Child Nutrition: The Achievable Imperative for Global Progress. New York: United Nations Publications; 2013. pp. 1-14

[3] Health Canada. 2013. Breastfeeeding in Canada. Available from: https://www150.statcan.gc.ca/n1/pub/82-624-x/2013001/article/11879-eng.htm [Accessed: 25 May 2020]

[4] Bai DL, Fong DY, Tarrant M. Factors associated with breastfeeding duration and exclusivity in mothers returning to paid employment postpartum. Maternal and Child Health Journal. 2015;**19**(5):990-999

[5] Lou Z, Zeng G, Huang L, Wang Y, Zhou L, Kavanagh KF. Maternal reported indicators and causes of insufficient milk supply. Journal of Human Lactation. 2014;**30**(4):466-473

[6] Braimoh J, Davies L. When 'breast' is no longer 'best': Post-partum constructions of infant-feeding in the hospital. Social Science & Medicine. 2014;**123**:82-89

[7] Abrams SA, Daniels SR. Protecting vulnerable infants by ensuring safe infant formula use. The Journal of Pediatrics. 2019;**211**:201-206

[8] Traves D. Understanding infant formula. Paediatrics and Child Health. 2019;**29**(9):384-388

[9] Lee E. Health, morality, and infant feeding: British mothers' experiences of formula milk use in the early weeks. Sociology of Health & Illness. 2007;**29**(7):1075-1090

[10] Lee E, Furedi F. Mothers' Experience of, and Attitudes to, Using Infant Formula in the Early Months. England: School of Social Policy, Sociology and Social Research, University of Kent. 2005. pp. 1-93

[11] Perez Locas C. Mechanism of formation of thermally generated potential toxicants in food related model systems [PhD thesis]. McGill University. 2008. Available from: https://escholarship.mcgill.ca/concern/theses/z890rx30j?locale=en [Accessed: 23 May 2020]

[12] Studer A, Blank I, Stadler RH. Thermal processing contaminants in foodstuffs and potential strategies of control. Czech Journal of Food Sciences. 2004;**22**(I):1

[13] Mogol BA, Gökmen V. Thermal process contaminants: Acrylamide, chloropropanols and furan. Current Opinion in Food Science. 2016;7:86-92

[14] National Institutes of Health (NIH). 2020. Available from: https://pubchem.ncbi.nlm.nih.gov/compound/Furan [Accessed: 20 May 2020]

[15] Becalski A, Seaman S. Furan precursors in food: A model study and development of a simple headspace method for determination of furan. Journal of AOAC International. 2005;**88**(1):102-106

[16] Perez Locas C, Yaylayan VA. Origin and mechanistic pathways of formation of the parent furan a food toxicant. Journal of Agricultural and Food Chemistry. 2004;**52**(22):6830-6836

[17] Joint, FAO, WHO Expert Committee on Food Additives World Health Organization. Safety Evaluation

of Certain Contaminants in Food: Prepared by the Seventy-Second Meeting of the Joint FAO/WHO Expert Committee on Food Additives (JECFA). 2011. Available from: https://apps.who.int/iris/bitstream/handle/10665/44520/9789241660631_eng.pdf [Accessed: 20 May 2020]

[18] National Toxicology Program. Toxicology and Carcinogenesis Studies of Furan (CAS No. 110-00-9) in F344 Rats and B6C3F1 Mice (Gavage Studies). Vol. 402. National Toxicology Program Technical Report Series; 1993. p. 1

[19] International Agency for Research on Cancer (IARC). Monographs on the Evaluation of Carcinogenic Risks to Humans. 1995. Available from: https://monographs.iarc.fr/list-of-classifications [Accessed: 20 May 2020]

[20] The US Food and Drug Administration (FDA). Exploratory Data on Furan in Food. 2004. Available from: https://www.fda.gov/food/chemicals/exploratory-data-furan-food [Accessed: 20 May 2020]

[21] The European Commission Recommendation. 2007/196/EC, on the Monitoring of the Presence of Furan in Foodstuffs. 2007. Available from: https://eur-lex.europa.eu/legal-content/EN/TXT/?uri=CELEX%3A32007H0196 [Accessed: 20 May 2020]

[22] Food and Agriculture Organization of the United Nations/World Health Organization (FAO/WHO). Joint FAO/WHO Expert Committee on Food Additives (JECFA) Rome Feb 2010: Furan. Technical Report Series 959/Food Additives Series 63. 2011. Available from: http://www.fao.org/3/a-at868e.pdf [Accessed: 20 May 2020]

[23] Crews C, Castle L. A review of the occurrence, formation and analysis of furan in heat-processed foods. Trends in Food Science & Technology. 2007;**18**(7):365-372

[24] Liu YT, Tsai SW. Assessment of dietary furan exposures from heat processed foods in Taiwan. Chemosphere. 2010;**79**(1):54-59

[25] European Food Safety Authority. Update on furan levels in food from monitoring years 2004-2010 and exposure assessment. EFSA Journal. 2011;**9**(9):2347

[26] Lambert M, Inthavong C, Desbourdes C, Hommet F, Sirot V, Leblanc JC, et al. Levels of furan in foods from the first French Total diet study on infants and toddlers. Food Chemistry. 2018;**266**:381-388

[27] EFSA Panel on Contaminants in the Food Chain (CONTAM), Knutsen HK, Alexander J, Barregård L, Bignami M, Brüschweiler B, et al. Risks for public health related to the presence of furan and methylfurans in food. EFSA Journal. 2017;**15**(10):e05005

[28] Health Canada. Furan. 2016. Available from: https://www.canada.ca/en/health-canada/services/food-nutrition/food-safety/chemical-contaminants/food-processing-induced-chemicals/furan.html [Accessed: 18 May 2020]

[29] Agence nationale de securit e sanitaire alimentation, environnement, travail (Anses). 2016. Etude de l'alimentation totale infantile. Available from: http://www.quasaprove.org/moodle/pluginfile.php/1421/mod_resource/content/1/EATi_Synth%C3%A8se%20et%20Conclusions.pdf [Accessed: 18 May 2020]

[30] Sirot V, Rivière G, Leconte S, Vin K, Traore T, Jean J, et al. French infant total diet study: Dietary exposure to heat-induced compounds (acrylamide, furan and polycyclic aromatic hydrocarbons) and associated health risks. Food and Chemical Toxicology. 2019;**130**:308-316

[31] Yau JCW, Kwong KP, Chung SWC, Ho YY, Xiao Y. Dietary exposure to

chloropropanols of secondary school students in Hong Kong. Food Additives and Contaminants: Part B Surveillance. 2008;**1**(2):93-99

[32] Seefelder W, Scholz G, Schilter B. Structural diversity of dietary fatty esters of chloropropanols and related substances. European Journal of Lipid Science and Technology. 2011;**113**(3):319-322

[33] Destaillats F, Craft BD, Sandoz L, Nagy K. Formation mechanisms of monochloropropanediol (MCPD) fatty acid diesters in refined palm (Elaeis guineensis) oil and related fractions. Food Additives & Contaminants: Part A. 2012;**29**(1):29-37

[34] Rahn AKK, Yaylayan VA. What do we know about the molecular mechanism of 3-MCPD ester formation? European Journal of Lipid Science and Technology. 2011;**113**(3):323-329

[35] Pudel F, Benecke P, Fehling P, Freudenstein A, Mattheaus B, Schwaf A. On the necessity of edible oil refining and possible sources of 3-MCPD and glycidyl esters. European Journal of Lipid Science and Technology. 2011;**113**(3):368e373

[36] The Joint Food and Agriculture Organization/World Health Organization Expert Committee on Food Additives. 3-Chloro-1,2-Propanediol. Safety Evaluation of Certain Food Additives and Contaminants. WHO Food Additives Series 48. Geneva: WHO; 2001

[37] The Joint Food and Agriculture Organization/World Health Organization Expert Committee on Food Additives. Sixty-Seventh Meeting – Summary and Conclusions. Rome: FAO; 2006. Available from: ftp://ftp.fao.org/ag/agn/jecfa/jecfa67_final.pdf [Accessed: 18 May 2020]

[38] Lee BQ, Khor SM. 3-Chloropropane-1, 2-diol (3-MCPD) in soy sauce: A review on the formation, reduction, and detection of this potential carcinogen. Comprehensive Reviews in Food Science and Food Safety. 2015;**14**(1):48-66

[39] Onami S, Cho YM, Toyoda T, Horibata K, Ishii Y, Umemura T, et al. Absence of in vivo genotoxicity of 3-monochloropropane-1, 2-diol and associated fatty acid esters in a 4-week comprehensive toxicity study using F344 gpt delta rats. Mutagenesis. 2014;**29**(4):295-302

[40] International Agency for Research on Cancer (IARC). Monographs on the Evaluation of Carcinogenic Risks to Humans. 2013. Available from: https://monographs.iarc.fr/list-of-classifications [Accessed: 21 May 2020]

[41] International Agency for Research on Cancer (IARC). 2013. Available from: https://monographs.iarc.fr/list-of-classifications [Accessed: 21 May 2020]

[42] International Agency for Research on Cancer (IARC). 2000. Available from: https://monographs.iarc.fr/list-of-classifications [Accessed: 21 May 2020]

[43] Andres S, Appel KE, Lampen A. Toxicology, occurrence and risk characterisation of the chloropropanols in food: 2-monochloro-1, 3-propanediol, 1, 3-dichloro-2-propanol and 2, 3-dichloro-1-propanol. Food and Chemical Toxicology. 2013;**58**:467-478

[44] European Food Safety Authority Panel on Contaminants in the Food Chain. Scientific opinion on the update of the risk assessment on 3-monochloropropane diol and its fatty acid esters. EFSA Journal. 2018;**16**(1):5083. Available from: https://efsa.onlinelibrary.wiley.com/doi/pdf/10.2903/j.efsa.2018.5083 [Accessed: 25 May 2020]

[45] Food Additives. Evaluation of Certain Contaminants in Food

(Eighty-Third Report of the Joint FAO/WHO Expert Committee on Food Additives). WHO Technical Report Series, No.1002; 2017

[46] FAO/WHO. Joint FAO/WHO Food Standards Programme-Codex Committee on Contaminants in Food. Discussion Paper on Chloropropanols Derived from the Manufacture of Acid-HVP and the Heat Processing of Foods. CX/CF 07/1/13. Rome: Codex Alimentarius Commission; 2007. Available from: http://www.fao.org/tempref/codex/Meetings/CCCF/cccf1/cf01_13e.pdf [Accessed: 25 May 2020]

[47] Food Standards Australia New Zealand (FSANZ). Chloropropanols in Food, an Analysis of the Public Health Risk, Technical Report Series No. 15. 2003. Available from: http://www.foodstandards.gov.au/_srcfiles/Chloropropanol%20Report%20%28no%20appendices%29-%2011%20Sep%2003b-2.pdf [Accessed: 25 May 2020]

[48] Hoogenboom LAP. Scientific opinion: Risks for human health related to the presence of 3-and 2-monochloropropanediol (MCPD), and their fatty acid esters, and glycidyl fatty acid esters in food. EFSA Journal. 2016;**14**(5):4426

[49] Wöhrlin F, Fry H, Lahrssen-Wiederholt M, Preiß-Weigert A. Occurrence of fatty acid esters of 3-MCPD, 2-MCPD and glycidol in infant formula. Food Additives & Contaminants: Part A. 2015;**32**(11):1810-1822

[50] Zelinková Z, Dolezal M, Velísek J. Occurrence of 3-chloropropane-1,2-diol fatty acid esters in infant and baby foods. European Food Research and Technology. 2009;**228**:571-578

[51] Weißhaar R. Fatty acid esters of 3-MCPD: Overview of occurrence and exposure estimates. European Journal of Lipid Science and Technology. 2011;**113**:304-308

[52] Spungen JH, MacMahon S, Leigh J, Flannery B, Kim G, Chirtel S, et al. Estimated US infant exposures to 3-MCPD esters and glycidyl esters from consumption of infant formula. Food Additives & Contaminants: Part A. 2018;**35**(6):1085-1092

[53] Arisseto AP, Silva WC, Scaranelo GR, Vicente E. 3-MCPD and glycidyl esters in infant formulas from the Brazilian market: Occurrence and risk assessment. Food Control. 2017;**77**:76-81

[54] National Institutes of Health (NIH). 2018. Available from: https://pubchem.ncbi.nlm.nih.gov/compound/acrylamide#section=Top [Accessed: 19 May 2020]

[55] Tareke E, Rydberg P, Karlsson P, Eriksson S, Tornqvist M. Analysis of acrylamide, a carcinogen formed in heated foodstuffs. Journal of Agricultural and Food Chemistry. 2002;**51**(17):4998-5006

[56] Stadler RH, Blank I, Varga N, Robert F, Hau J, Guy PA, et al. Food chemistry: Acrylamide from Maillard reaction products. Nature. 2002;**419**(6906):449-450

[57] Guenther H, Anklam E, Wenzl T, Stadler RH. Acrylamide in coffee: Review of progress in analysis. Formation and level reduction. Food Additives and Contaminants. 2007;**24**(1):60-70

[58] National Toxicology Program (NTP). NTP Technical Report on the Toxicology and Carcinogenesis. Studies of Glycidamide (CAS No. 5694-00-8) in F344/N Nctr Rats and B6C3F1/Nctr Mice (Drinking Water Studies). NTP TR 588. National Institutes of Health. Public Health Service. U.S. Department of Health and Human Services; 2014.

Available from: http://ntp.niehs.nih.gov/ntp/htdocs/lt_rpts/tr588_508.pdf [Accessed: 19 May 2020]

[59] Von Tungeln LS, Doerge DR, da Costa GG, Matilde Marques M, Witt WM, Koturbash I, et al. Tumorigenicity of acrylamide and its metabolite glycidamide in the neonatal mouse bioassay. International Journal of Cancer. 2012;**131**:2008-2015

[60] Kadawathagedara M, Botton J, de Lauzon-Guillain B, Meltzer HM, Alexander J, Brantsaeter AL, et al. Dietary acrylamide intake during pregnancy and postnatal growth and obesity: Results from the Norwegian mother and child cohort study (MoBa). Environment International. 2018;**113**:325-334

[61] Goffeng LO, Alvestrand M, Ulvestad B, Sorensen KA, Skaug V, Kjuus H. Self-reported symptoms and neuropsychological function among tunnel workers previously exposed to acrylamide and N-methylolacrylamide. Scandinavian Journal of Work, Environment and Health. 2011;**37**:136-146

[62] Wilson KM, Mucci LA, Rosner BA, Willett WC. A prospective study of dietary acrylamide intake and the risk of breast, endometrial, and ovarian cancers. Cancer Epidemiology, Biomarkers & Prevention. 2010;**19**(10):2503-2515

[63] Hirvonen T, Kontto J, Jestoi M, Valsta L, Peltonen K, Pietinen P, et al. Dietary acrylamide intake and the risk of cancer among Finnish male smokers. Cancer Causes & Control. 2010;**21**(12):2223-2229

[64] Liu ZM, Tse LA, Ho SC, Wu S, Chen B, Chan D, et al. Dietary acrylamide exposure was associated with increased cancer mortality in Chinese elderly men and women: A 11-year prospective study of Mr. and Ms. OS Hong Kong. Journal of Cancer Research and Clinical Oncology. 2017;**143**(11):2317-2326

[65] Mucci LA, Sandin S, Bälter K, Adami HO, Magnusson C, Weiderpass E. Acrylamide intake and breast cancer risk in Swedish women. JAMA. 2005;**293**(11):1322-1327

[66] Schouten LJ, Hogervorst JG, Konings EJ, Goldbohm RA, van den Brandt PA. Dietary acrylamide intake and the risk of head-neck and thyroid cancers: Results from the Netherlands cohort study. American Journal of Epidemiology. 2009;**170**(7):873-884

[67] Kotemori A, Ishihara J, Zha L, Liu R, Sawada N, Iwasaki M, et al. Dietary acrylamide intake and the risk of endometrial or ovarian cancers in Japanese women. Cancer Science. 2018;**109**(10):3316-3325

[68] International Agency for Research on Cancer (IARC). 1994. Available from: https://monographs.iarc.fr/list-of-classifications [Accessed: 21 May 2020]

[69] EFSA Panel on Contaminants in the Food Chain (CONTAM). Scientific opinion on acrylamide in food. EFSA Journal. 2015;**13**(6):4104

[70] Fohgelberg P, Rosén J, Hellenäs KE, Abramsson-Zetterberg L. The acrylamide intake via some common baby food for children in Sweden during their first year of life—An improved method for analysis of acrylamide. Food and Chemical Toxicology. 2005;**43**(6):951-959

[71] Elias A, Roasto M, Reinik M, Nelis K, Nurk E, Elias T. Acrylamide in commercial foods and intake by infants in Estonia. Food Additives & Contaminants: Part A. 2017;**34**(11):1875-1884

[72] Mojska H, Gielecińska I, Stoś K. Determination of acrylamide level

in commercial baby foods and an assessment of infant dietary exposure. Food and Chemical Toxicology. 2012;**50**(8):2722-2728

[73] Health Canada. Health Canada's Revised Exposure Assessment of Acrylamide in Food. Bureau of Chemical Safety. Food Directorate. Health Products and Food Branch; 2012. pp. 1-19. Available from: https://www.canada.ca/content/dam/hc-sc/migration/hc-sc/fn-an/alt_formats/pdf/securit/chem-chim/food-aliment/acrylamide/rev-eval-exposure-exposition-eng.pdf [Accessed: 15 May 2020]

[74] Shen H, Guan R, Ding G, Chen Q, Lou X, Chen Z, et al. Polychlorinated dibenzo-p-dioxins/furans (PCDD/Fs) and polychlorinated biphenyls (PCBs) in Zhejiang foods (2006-2015): Market basket and polluted areas. Science of the Total Environment. 2017;**574**:120-127

[75] Schuhmacher M, Mari M, Nadal M, Domingo JL. Concentrations of dioxins and furans in breast milk of women living near a hazardous waste incinerator in Catalonia, Spain. Environment International. 2019;**125**:334-341

[76] Sörgel F, Weissenbacher R, Kinzig-Schippers M, Hofmann A, Illauer M, Skott A, et al. Acrylamide: Increased concentrations in homemade food and first evidence of its variable absorption from food, variable metabolism and placental and breast milk transfer in humans. Chemotherapy. 2002;**48**(6):267-274

[77] Zelinková Z, Novotný O, Schůrek J, Velíšek J, Hajšlová J, Doležal M. Occurrence of 3-MCPD fatty acid esters in human breast milk. Food Additives & Contaminants: Part A. 2008;**25**:669-676

[78] Jędrkiewicz R, Głowacz-Różyńska A, Gromadzka J, Kloskowski A, Namieśnik J. Indirect determination of MCPD fatty acid esters in lipid fractions of commercially available infant formulas for the assessment of infants' health risk. Food Analytical Methods. 2016;**9**(12):3460-3469

[79] van den Berg M, Kypke K, Kotz A, Tritscher A, Lee SY, Magulova K, et al. WHO/UNEP global surveys of PCDDs, PCDFs, PCBs and DDTs in human milk and benefit–risk evaluation of breastfeeding. Archives of Toxicology. 2017;**91**(1):83-96

[80] Costopoulou D, Vassiliadou I, Papadopoulos A, Makropoulos V, Leondiadis L. Levels of dioxins, furans and PCBs in human serum and milk of people living in Greece. Chemosphere. 2006;**65**(9):1462-1469

[81] van Leeuwen FR, Feeley M, Schrenk D, Larsen JC, Farland W, Younes M. Dioxins: WHO's tolerable daily intake (TDI) revisited. Chemosphere. 2000;**40**(9-11):1095-1101

[82] Focant JF, Fréry N, Bidondo ML, Eppe G, Scholl G, Saoudi A, et al. Levels of polychlorinated dibenzo-p-dioxins, polychlorinated dibenzofurans and polychlorinated biphenyls in human milk from different regions of France. Science of the Total Environment. 2013;**452**:155-162

[83] Huang R, Wang P, Zhang J, Chen S, Zhu P, Huo W, et al. The human body burden of polychlorinated dibenzo-p-dioxins/furans (PCDD/Fs) and dioxin-like polychlorinated biphenyls (DL-PCBs) in residents' human milk from Guangdong Province, China. Toxicology Research. 2019;**8**(4):552-559